Understanding Traditional Chinese Medicine

Culture and Knowledge

Edited by Friedrich G. Wallner

Vol. 10

PETER LANG

Frankfurt am Main · Berlin · Bern · Bruxelles · New York · Oxford · Wien

Friedrich G. Wallner
Gertrude Kubiena
Martin J. Jandl
(eds.)

Understanding Traditional Chinese Medicine

Consultant: Lena Springer

PETER LANG
Internationaler Verlag der Wissenschaften

Bibliographic Information published by the Deutsche Nationalbibliothek
The Deutsche Nationalbibliothek lists this publication in the Deutsche Nationalbibliografie; detailed bibliographic data is available in the internet at <http://www.d-nb.de>.

Printed with financial support of the
Federal Ministry of Science and Research in Vienna.

BM.W_Fª

Bundesministerium für Wissenschaft und Forschung

This volume emerges from the project
"Comparative Analysis of Central Expressions of Traditional
Chinese Medicine in the Context of Modern Western Medicine"
financed by MedChin.

Cover illustration:
"Nike von Samothraki"
Courtesy of Kovac-Verlag.

ISSN 1613-902X
ISBN 978-3-631-56709-8

Table of Contents

Preface

The 2007 Beijing Workshop *Comparative Analysis of Important Expressions of TCM in Context with Modern Western Medicine* was an outstanding project. It was part of the 20 years jubilee celebration of MedChin, an Austrian non profit organization for TCM postgraduate training outside China. It was an outstanding TCM event because there was no pressure on time, by financial interests of the medical industry. In this relaxed atmosphere three scientists from Austria had the unique opportunity to discuss the subject for two weeks with famous Chinese scientists and TCM practitioners under the guidance of Prof. Zhang Qicheng in the pleasant atmosphere of the Swissotel. For me the astonishing output has several aspects.

Concerning TCM terminology my starting point was originally the facilitation of acceptance by Western TCM students, based on understanding. The very different interpretation of classical texts and modern textbooks of TCM are severe obstacles aggravating the persisting cultural difference, the intruding into a different world of thinking.

During the workshop it turned out that in China TCM terminology is a very actual topic and even more emphasized on than in the West. The difficulties of understanding, teaching and "digesting" TCM are not a specific problem of the Western world but as well of Chinese teachers and students. The manifoldness of the interpretation of many TCM terms is not only generated by translation into foreign languages, but is as well based on the difficulties of transferring classical into modern Chinese, the multiplicity of the meaning of one single character/word and on the change of meaning in the course of historical development. As a result of neglecting the historical development we are sometimes confused by various interpretations of TCM key terms: Some ideas behind various key expressions have changed their meaning in the course of time as well as under the influence from abroad, e.g. cultural transfer of religion, science and technology. Still more momentous: "The standardization of terms of TCM became one of the keys for the modernization and internationalization of TCM" (as Prof Zhu Jianping said on May 4th 2007) in China. These items are considered vital necessities for the survival of TCM. Strange enough: While Chinese Medicine becomes gradually established outside China, it strugges for survival inside China, against the mighty lobbying of modern Western Medicine. In China there are great efforts to modernize and standardize TCM-terminology in order to internationalize and preserve TCM. Investigation on these topics is supported generously by the government. Although a great part of the work is already done, a comprehensive result still lacks. One great project, titled "TCM Masters Knowledge Mining", deals with systemic analysis as a kind of meta-synthesis of 100 TCM masters' knowledge. One of the problems is the lacking readiness for collaboration between the old masters.

The National Committee for Examination and Definition of Scientific and Technological Terms researches on a national project in several three- respectively five-years-projects, covering all scientific and technological fields. Traditional Chinese Medicine is one of the several items (about 60). Some of the leading personalities of the TCM-project, into which the Chinese Academy of Science is involved, took part in our workshop and gave most valuable contributions.

In spite of these serious efforts, up to now there is no unified concept in China how to deal with the translation of TCM key terms – literally or interpretive. An argument for interpretive translation is the easier understanding outside and inside China; arguments for literal translation are the possibility of re-translation and of enabling the users to read and understand various classical books. I personally opt for literal translation with connotations.

Since the 19th century there has been a tendency to submit TCM to modern Western medicine, concerning terminology as well as research methodology. Several times the government even tried to "annul and abolish" TCM considering it an "obstacle", e.g. the edict from 1929, which was encountered successfully by TCM practitioners (17 March 1929). In 2000, during the TCM World Congress in Beijing, almost every speaker emphasized the importance of 'proving' TCM by application of Western methodology.

Up to recent times the mainstream of the current theory of science allowed only one truth, suggesting: If modern Western Medicine is true, TCM cannot be true. The theory of constructive realism encounters this thesis, emphasizing on the possibility of the co-existence of apparently contradictory systems respectively realities. Constructive realism represented by Wallner can be seen as the theoretical foundation for a new tendency coming up in China after the beginning of the 3rd Millennium – growing self-consciousness with regard to Chinese thinking and Chinese methodology.

Chinese Medicine can only be practiced and investigated successfully if Chinese thinking and methodology are applied. Of course, modern medicinal knowledge must not be neglected. In contrary, it has to be considered very carefully. But sometimes Chinese Medicine is simply more rapid and more effective than modern Western Medicine. This is because Modern Western Medicine can treat a disease only of the origin – in the modern sense – is known. TCM treats the obvious "pattern", what can be experienced by the human sense organs.

E.g. SARS: The pathogen – in the Western sense of meaning – and as a follow up a relatively uncertain method of prevention (vaccination) was finally found two years after the first occurrence of SARS. Prescriptions of Chinese Medicine were very successful, but only if applied in accordance with Chinese thinking, including environmental influences, individual constitution and condition etc. Applied by Western MDs without this knowledge, simplified and reduced to one standard prescription – as the excluding Western thinking requires – TCM prescriptions failed. The manifoldness of the individual Chinese prescriptions and herbs – each of them about 100 and more – was considered an impediment for scientific acknowledgement of the method. Nevertheless investigation on TCM with modern Western methodology has to be continued to give certainty to Western appliers. There should be serious efforts to publish the results of PR China's governmental projects on TCM-terminology immediately in English and German.

A strange experience was that it was not quite easy for our Chinese friends to realize that a project is a project, even if it is not organized or sponsored by the government but more or less is a private project. They only understood the given structure when I told them the story of the early Austrian Himalaya expeditions: If somebody was able on his own to pay for travel, permissions, Sherpas, porters, equipment etc. some people said: "This is not an expedition because it is not sponsored and organized by one of the official mountaineer's associations". Nevertheless it was an expedition because the target was the exploration of an unknown region. This is valid as well for the 2007 Beijing TCM workshop.

Many new projects were created by the Beijing workshop 2007 but it is not easy to find sponsors for investigation in basics of TCM. The public interest emphasizes on the bargain of import-export of Chinese drugs and herbs. This becomes obvious by studying the schedules of actual international TCM congresses. The fact that Chinese Medicine outside China only can be spread successfully if the basics are understandable and digestible for Western students is neglected. China can close its herbal shops for the West if the Western practitioners don't get an optimal TCM education.

Finally I want to express my cordial thanks to all of the participants of the workshop, first of all to the leader of the Chinese group Zhang Qicheng, and the hope that they enjoyed it – as I did in spite of a broken clavicle. Please see the acknowledgements. And please let us continue such relaxed discussions on TCM! Last not least thanks for the friendship and the friendliness of our Chinese partners, for the gratification of their precious time for a subject, which must appear very banal to them.

Prof. Dr. med et Mag. phil. Dr. Gertrude Kubiena
Mallorca (Spain), in January 2008

Lu Guangxin

The fundamental principles of traditional Chinese medicine

Translated by Lin Tingxiu

Medicine (World III) is a spiritual product accumulated through long-term historical experience which is the result of the interaction between the world workers (World II) and medical objects (World I). The Gentlemen value fundamental principles from which Tao originates. Tao, in the theory of Chinese medicine, comes from fundamental principles which are the research objects and aims of practice. From the point of view of Popper's [1] three worlds, it is the historical and spiritual products (World III) of the interaction between Chinese medicine professionals (World II) who are the main body of cognition and practice and actual objects (World I) which Chinese medicine studies. Only valuing fundament principles can guarantee Tao. Actual objects (I) [2] are the study objects of Chinese medicine which is basis for the existence of Chinese medicine professionals (II) and the development of Chinese medical theories (III). The cognition and practice of Chinese medicine professionals start from Tao and Chinese medical theories are the theoretical model that continuously pushes it close to the actual study objects. Therefore, the object and aim of Chinese medicine is the root and Chinese medicine and its theories are the branches. If root (the patient) and branches (the doctor) are not harmonious, the evil will slip in and vise versa. Chinese medicine is in a large environment of modern science and modern medicine. So, what will it face?

---

1   Karl Popper (1902-1994), born in Austria, British scientific philosopher and political philosopher
2   Research objects of Chinese medicine is mutual conversion process of health and disease brought by the interaction between human and environment, which means the research objects are not confined to diseases. The process of diagnosis in Chinese medicine is to understand the gradual conversion of health and disease through the interaction between human and environment. The practice of preserving one's health and treating diseases is to affect this process.

1. Potential crisis of medicine

According to the survey data of WHO (the World Health Organisation), among the factors that affect human health and longevity, how much does modern medicine account for? The answer reads: 8 per cent. Except that, genetic factor accounts for 15 per cent, climate 7 per cent, social factor 10 per cent, individual factors like personal life and psychological state 60 per cent. What does this mean? First-class medical facilities and health care and 100 per cent efforts only occupy 8 per cent. Because of the uneven distribution of medical service, hard-to-get-treated becomes a problem which unprecedentedly declines the social trust in medicine, hospitals and doctors and triggers a contemporary global health crisis.

In 1977 the theory that medical model should be converted into bio-psycho-social medicine was proposed. Since 1993 the international community, including China, has raised a hot discussion about the purposes of medicine. In 2005 the health care reform issue induced a hot debate. But unfortunately, these two issues did not impact each other after they entered China. They are discussed as two isolated issues and two concepts, which is not enough.

For decades, at abroad, the problem about medical models and medical purposes should raise our reflection about traditional medicine. Why does the contemporary global medical crisis exist? Why does the western world discuss medical models and medical purposes? It can be said that contemporary global medical crisis rooted in modern medical model which mainly aims at techniques that can cure diseases. In conclusion, this is caused by long-term medicalization of medical mistakes.

2. Relationship between medicine and science

In *Confession of a Medical Heretic* (《一个医学判逆者的自白》) Mendelson[1] (1980) claimed: "How to defend our own lives from traps of doctors, chemical drugs and hospitals." On the front cover he sets out five points: (1) annual physical examination is a trap; (2) hospitals are the places with

---

1   Robert S. Mendelson (1926-1988), American MD, leader of American Medical Association, president of American Alliance for Health. In 1980, he published his masterpiece *Confession of a Medical Heretic*.

danger and death for patients; (3) for most of the surgery, injury is more than benefit; (4) tests and checkouts are unreasonable and full of flaws; (5) most chemicals are the reasons of causing and adding diseases. Mendelson also thought that the self-claimed scientific allopathy was very non-scientific, scientific superstition and superstition in the cloak of science.

What are the relations between medicine and science? Is there a medical scientification or a scientific medicalization?

2.1 Medical scientification

The signs of modern medical scientification are that medical practice (take TCM as an example) – how to treat diseases – has been converted into the understanding of diseases (take western medicine as an example) – given in the question 'Where does diseases come from?' The relationship between these two is shown in the tabel on the next page.

Modern medical scientification learns from natural science's objectified thinking of materialistic epistemology and its cognitive direction-backward, downward and outward. Backward means structure-analyzing epistemology exploding its origination-how it comes. Downward means micro-entities essence and components theory-what compose of a disease. Outward means linear determinism of cause and effect-how a disease comes and how it should be cured. This is a kind of objectist epistemology in the concept of scientific knowledge.

2.2 Medicine should not worship the ground science treads on

Engels[1] once said as long as the natural sciences thought, their development would be expressed as hypothesis. In other words, science is actually a kind of theoretical hypothesis about objective things. After tested by practice, hypothesis becomes a science.

Medical practice (take Chinese medicine as an example)	Understanding of diseases (take western medicine as an example)
intentional thinking of humanism	objectified thinking of materialistic epistemology
forward, upward and inward thinking-inducing direction	backward, downward and outward cognitive direction
practice-how to cure diseases	understanding-where diseases come from
integrated system of life in creative practice	analysis of material entity structure in understanding
spirit and qi respond inside	linear determinism of cause and effect
self-organ evolutionary regulation	chemical substance basis
make efforts to explore and enhance	make efforts to find out diseases and get rid of them completely
auto-regulation	pathogenic factors
resistant reaction	pathological damage
circumstantial change	spatial orientation
practical medical model with human health as ecological objectives	biomedical medical model targeted at diseases based on explanations of physical and chemical principles

If we consider medical purposes and medical models as unification, medicine is a kind of practice. Physicians govern, but govern what? Govern

---

1   Engels Friedrich (1820-1895), German socialist philosopher

things to make them orderly. What is governance? Control water, scholarship, country and home, all of which is a process of governance, and governance is management. Western management guru said management was not a science. But science can provide management services so management does not affiliate to any science. What kind of science, do you think, medicine belongs to? Astronomy? Geography? No. Science is knowledge of a certain field and is a categorized study on one kind of the nonego material world. Strictly speaking, science is only about the scientific knowledge of epistemology. However, medicine is practice and practice is not science.

Our crisis lies in that medicine worships the ground science treads on. Modern western science is a science of matter, which means it is a science composed of nonego materials. Its cognitive direction is to understand and solve problems backward, downward and outward. ›Backward‹ means to probe into its origin, how it comes from. ›Downward‹ means components theory, what a disease is composed of. ›Outward‹ means linear theory of cause and effect, how a disease comes and how to cure it.

If everything is like that, medicine would be twisted. The cause of the wrongness is treating functional aims of medicine, part of the research objects-disease and theoretical explanation on diseases as science. So I think that modern medicine can be summed up in these words: make efforts to find out diseases and clear them up. It has indeed done a lot of work but unfortunately only accounts for 8 per cent effects among other factors.

In 1978 we have experienced a hot discussion about the truth of scientific epistemology. This time: discussion on the criterion of truth and the restoration of the authority of practice should be able to be universally applied to medical field. Feyerabend hinted: "Success can be achieved by using non-scientific strength to overcome the resistance of science." This is the necessary prerequisite why we need a great ideological emancipation to reconstruct ecological medicine for human health.

Ecological medicine for human health should be able to achieve exceeding and tolerating natural science as holding the world with virtue and keeping harmony in diversity. Allopathy as the strong point of diseases-focused medicine should be restricted and promoted to a higher level like appropriately using poisons to cure diseases and avoiding harming healthy qi, eating certain kind of food can tonify healthy qi but for too long can also cause diseases, no evil, no development and no evil, no speed.

Science should be able to serve the healthy medical development; it must put the human beings better life and development at the first place. Medical scientification is a mistake but scientific medicalization is the right way.

3. Healthy medicine

3.1 Times call for health

In 1993 International Research Plans of Medical Purpose (《医学的目的国际研究计划》) sharply pointed out: "Contemporary global medical crisis rooted in modern medical model which mainly aims at the techniques that can cure diseases and rules the medical world." However, WHO, in the report of *Meet the 21st Century Challenge* (《迎接 21 世纪的挑战》), pointed out: "The 21st century medicine should not continuously focus on research about diseases but on human health as the main medical research direction."

This is because since Carson[1] issued *Silent Spring* (《寂静的春天》) in 1962, in which he revealed direct confrontation and direct complement represented by pesticides and fertilisers respectively, bringing about chemical pollution and ecological destruction to mankind and the environment. When we reflect on medicine, it is discovered that in the past 100 years chemotherapy with large-scale use of chemical synthesized drugs has caused drug-related chemical pollution and human body has constantly been impacted by chemicals, which has produced long-term adverse consequences and even opposite effect against the purposes of treatment:

Anti-metabolic chemical therapy aimed at eliminating pathogeny brings about multiple resistances to drugs very soon. On the one hand, it speeds up the process that drugs fall into disuse, adds difficulties in the development of new drugs and increases cost. On the other hand, it accelerates the variability of pathogens and creates new pathogens and new diseases retarder for changing pathological receptors or channels are

1   Rachel Carson (1907-1964), American writer

widely used to correct pathological hyperfunction, but receptors become hypersensitive and drug dependence increases which means when the drug is stopped the disease will come again and even become worse. This can also increase inner environmental shocks and chronic changes and recurrence.

Targeted chemical drugs aimed at removing focus are used, which intensifies internal chemical pollution, overloads antigens and causes immune response errors and increases immune hypersensitivity and auto-immune diseases. Direct exogenous confrontation leads to endogenous priming action: direct exogenous complement leads to endogenous function inhibition. In recent decades, human peripheral leukocyte count has decreased by more than 1/3 and male sperm count and activity dropped significantly.

The chemical field also realized the ponderance and ultimacy of this problem so they brought forward green chemistry and the concept of environment-friendly chemistry and developed combinatorial chemistry technology with a view to meet ecological requirements for adapting to human beings and the living environment.

Times are calling for changes in medical models. Psychological and social factors only exist in humans, so the medical model can be converted from biomedical to physianthropy. The modernization of medicine needs a constructive and aggressive medicine. Here the nature of medicine needs to be understood again. Since people become the main medical objects, then we should reveal the nature of medical function by understanding people and prescribe development rules of modern medicine.

Development trend of modern medicine will be:

- from chemical level based on materials to life level seeking for self-evolution and target regulation
- from biology to physianthropy
- curing-disease medicine to health medicine
- from confronting medicine to ecological medicine

3.2 Chinese medicine is non-scientific

Medicine is not a scientific epistemology about material world rather than people. It is a kind of practice targeted at people and for their health. Chinese medicine considers its objects as a self-organizing-and-evolving regulating system. Human beings' behaviors are adaptive stress response, which is self-organized.

Chinese medicine is non-scientific because it is not like the western material science which understands external things and solves problems backward, downward and outward, but is functional target dynamics which is a forward, upward and inward self-organizing-and-evolving regulating system.

Feyerabend[1] once said that Chinese government promoted traditional medicine and made diversification possible for medical advancement. Here he particularly stressed that medical development was diversified development not the so-called scientific monism and egoism. But he added that this could only be achieved when non-scientific strength broke the resistance of science.

3.3 Where to go-Chinese medicine

In the late 19th and early 20th century Liang Qichao[2] commented on Chinese medicine. He said Chinese medicine could cure diseases but no one could tell how. Chen Duxiu[3] also said that Chinese medicine did not know science. There are three reasons: without anatomy, body structure can not be known; drug property analysis, that is physical and chemical analysis, is not done; bacterial viruses are not understood. Hu Shi[4] said that western medicine could clearly explain what the disease was and where it ca-

---

1 Paul Feyerabend (1924-1994), Austrian philosopher and historian of science
2 Liang Qichao, 1876-1929, courtesy name, Zhuoru, pseudonym, Rengong, alias, Bingshizhuren, born in Xinhui, Guangdong Province, modern politician and litterateur, a student of Kang Youwei. They two,called *Kangliang*, adovocated The Reform Movement of 1898
3 Chen Duxiu, 1880 -1942, courtesy name, Zhongfu, one of the three founders of China's Communist Party
4 Hu Shi, 1891-1962, courtesy name, Shizhi, born in Jixi, Anhui Province, modern scholar, thinker and famous character in cultural movement in China.

me from. Western medicine can clearly describe etiology, pathology and the location of diseases so even if it can not cure diseases, it is scientific but Chinese medicine can cure diseases, only because it can not clearly explain diseases, and it is unscientific. Therefore, the so-called unscientific Chinese medicine can cure diseases but can not explain them. Then, why does Chinese medicine can cure and prevent diseases without understanding them?

Chinese medicine stresses on an ideal state which is ecological harmony and evolution. This ideal state is very important because it can avoid harm and get benefit for us. In *Zhou Li* (《周礼》) it is asked what the physician's responsibility is, giving the answer: Making poison serve for medicine which means turning poison into medicinal drugs to benefit people. As early as 2000 years ago, Bangu gave Chinese medicine a definition: Chinese medicine is a tool to heal the wounded and rescue the dying. In other words, Chinese medicine is a method, a technique and a tool serving for humankind, their healthy development and evolution.

Chinese medicine considers humans as self-organizing-and-evolving regulating systems and their behaviors are adaptive stress responses. The ability of and efforts made by Chinese medicine on understanding and eliminating diseases are not enough. Its task is to explore and develop. But explore what? Explore resisting and self defending ability and self-regulating ability in self-organizing-and-evolving regulating system. Discover these abilities, develop them and rely on them to help people to achieve better practical results.

Chinese medicine is people oriented. First it starts from people and second it is for people. Starting from people means as a doctor, his objects are conscious people. In the past century Chinese medicine has withstood all kinds of disasters, resulting in almost being eliminated but with Chinese herbs kept. Here doctors cut no ice and that which can cure diseases is medicine and technology. I think modern western medicine takes the same road which means the doctors and medicine step down and only drugs are preserved. The doctors only see the examination results and then prescribe drugs. The objects are no longer people but some indexes. No wonder WHO said that modern medical care accounted only for 8 per cent among all the factors that effect human health and longevity. Chinese medicine considers for curing and preventing diseases 30 per cent depends on medicine and 70 per cent depends on patients themselves. I think this is reasonable.

In 1908 experiments done by Ehrlich[1], Nobel Prize winner in Medicine, Germany physician and immunologist, showed that for treating trypanosomiasis with trypan red, the real dose to cure the infected animals was only 1/6 of the laboratory dose. Where did the other 5/6 come from? This is a major medical proposition and can only be understood as self-healing functions of organisms.

The cause of SARS is virus. The whole world is in hot pursuit of the virus, but if we find the virus, will we be able to find a solution? Bird flu killed more than 100 people around the world, but in order to prevent bird flu, 150 million birds have died or been killed. Is this really worthy? Is this scientific? Chinese medicine stresses all that are invaded by evils are lacking of healthy qi so the existence of virus is not the ultimate reason.

Chinese medicine considers doctors as lower curer. Upper doctors govern the country and build it into an environment-friendly and harmonious society. Chinese Medicine treats people (people' mind-set and stability) as its objects. Lower doctors cure diseases and in this level, Chinese medicine and western medicine are equal. Chinese medicine does not know pathogen, pathology and location of diseases but it studies abilities of defending and resisting diseases, regulating and self-organizing that means unity of spirit, qi and the body.

The purpose of medicine is to provide service for human health and ecological harmony. Medicine is a creative practice for life. We can create wedging effect by adding in doctor's initiative. We can produce additive effect by mobilising surrounding environment. In short, make the end of practice better than the beginning and bring about spillover effect. Doctor's practice is to work hard to make the end better than the starting point. I think it is justified why Chinese medicine can survive when being accused of unscientific and be internationalized.

---

1   Paul Ehrlich (1854-1915), German physician, bacteriologist and one of the founders of modern chemotherapy

4. Chinese medicine – where to go?

In the author's preface, Zhang Zhongjing[1] of Eastern Han dynasty said: "Learn from ancient wisdom and various fields." Lu Yuanlei[2] of modern times pointed out: "Promote ancient knowledge and combine mew knowledge." In 1959 Zhang Cigong[3] pointed out: "In order for integration, first it has to seek independence." As the saying goes: "Practice is more important than only reading." In 1929 Zhang Taiyan[4] stressed: "Patients themselves are the best teachers for doctors."

Where should Chinese medicine go?

Objectively speaking, there are some diseases that Chinese medicine can not cure. Chinese medicine is not a panacea just like western medicine. As previously mentioned the function of Chinese medicine accounts for 30 per cent and the real cure of diseases is self-regulating ability. The way for Chinese medicine is summed up as: holding world with virtue, keeping harmony in diversity, constantly striving to become stronger, exceeding and tolerating.

---

1   Zhang Zhongjing (AD 25-220), distinguished medical scientist in Eastern Han Dynasty, known as medical saint. His works were compiled into two books *Treatise on Cold-induced Febrile Diseases* and *Synopsis of Golden Chamber.*
2   Lu Yuan Lei (1894-1955), courtesy name, Pengnian, born in Chuansha County, Jiangsu province, modern physician. He learned and converged Chinese and western medicine and is one of the representatives of school of conbination of chinese and western medicine.
3   Zhang Cigong (1903~1959), courtesy name, Chengzhi, pseudonym Zhian, born in Zhenjiang, Jiangsu Province, is an outstanding modern educator, clinical doctor and innovator of Chinese medicine.
4   Zhang Taiyan (1869-1936), courtesy name, Binglin, pseudonym, Taiyan, born in Yuhang, Zhejiang Province. He is a democratic revolutionist, thinker and famous scholar during late Qing Dynasty and early Repubic of China. His studies involve history, philosophy, and politics and so on and he wrote a lot of works.

Fritz Wallner & Florian Schmidsberger

How to research TCM?

1. Leading question and problem: the way of researching TCM

This text focuses on two questions concerning the research on Traditional Chinese Medicine (TCM) as well as the scientific approach of this research.

First we want to ask: What have we to do if we want to research TCM adequately? – To explain this question: If we research on TCM and attempt to know its concepts, its system, its structure, its theoretical fundaments and especially its typical way of thinking and healing we have to raise the question of how to manage this. We have to question what we have to do if want to be effective on the one hand and to do a correct research on TCM on the other hand – what means to achieve an improved understanding of TCM and its typical and genuine way of being science.

Second we question: In what way do we have to approach to TCM if we consider the relation of Occidental and far-east science? – To explain this question we want to start with a famous research program that was recently carried out in Germany and that reflects a wide spread idea of dealing with the system of TCM. This German studies were emphasizing the question about the efficiency of acupuncture. They formed three groups: the first one underwent the treatment of Western Medicine, the second group the treatment of real acupuncture while the third group was treated by pseudo-acupuncture what means that the doctor takes the needle but sticks the wrong spots. – And what was the result? First the Western treatment was worse than the Chinese treatment in this field in all cases. And second there is no big difference in the efficiency of the real acupuncture and the pseudo-acupuncture.

Now we could deduce from this: The theory of acupuncture is nonsense and absurd or what ever you do is better than Western medicine. But what do we find here? This study states that both medicines can be compared without any considerations, that both can be treated in an equate way, that the concept of placebo can be applied and used in both medical systems. In opposition to these allegated presuppositions we raise the question whether it is really possible to compare the systems of Occidental and traditional Chinese medicine? And whether we really can assume that both systems are compatible? – Based on the results of the research and developed ideas in the field of philosophy of science we have to reject these theses. We have to state that – as we are going to give reasons for later in this text[1] – it is not possible to equate both medical systems, to assume that both can be treated in the same way, that both are compatible.

Thus if we want to research on TCM, we also and especially have to consider the approach to TCM and to reflect of how to deal with this systems? We have to ask for the relation of TCM and the currently important Occidental medicine. We have to ask in which way we have to refer to TCM? – That's our second question. It should be obvious that the first question is connected with the second one and goes back to it. That means that if we want to do a TCM-adequate research (one that is done effectively and correctly) we also and especially have to consider of how to approach to TCM – and that's how both questions are connected.

Based on the named questions and the given explanations we can say what this text is about: the following reasoning and attempts to answer the two questions are to consider as preconsiderations for a TCM-adequate research as well as reflections of the approach of researching TCM. That means that our argumentation is not to consider as showing up concrete results on the research of TCM and its ways and concepts of healing. Instead it has to be understood as a methodological reflection. If we think of the classic differentiation of content and form we can characterise our arguments as concerning the form of the research on TCM.

To answer the questions this text is going to combine the research on TCM with concepts and ideas coming from the field of philosophy of science. These concepts and ideas shall be used to enlighten the relation of the two different systems of medicine respectively the two different systems of scientific thinking. They shall be used to explain the differences of those two systems as well as their typical way of thinking.

---

1   see chapter 2.2

To answer the questions – what is going to happen in part B – we will take three steps: Firstly, we will state the ideas of Constructive Realism to solve the named problems and questions concerning the research on TCM. There we will give an impression in what direction the position of Constructive Realism will take us and which ideas will be central for solving the questions. Secondly, we are bound to give an explanation and to give reasons for this concept of research as it is described in the first step. Thus we are going to show you the main concepts and ideas of the position of Constructive Realism that are used to answer the questions. In that respect we are going to explain its central aims (to understand its position), its concept of science, its methodology to become aware of the typical way of thinking of a system as well as its concept of scientific knowledge.As a third step we finally will give concrete insights into the relation of the two scientific systems. There we want to apply the named concepts of Constructive Realism, their concepts of science and knowledge as well its typical methodology on the research of TCM. In that respect we are going to characterise the typical way of the thinking of Western science and TCM including their differences. Finally we are going to name some advices for the research on TCM as well as some mistakes that may occur and that should be avoided.

2. Ideas to solve the scientific problems: reflecting the approach

2.1 The proposal of "Constructive Realism"

Let us reconsider the central questions and issue of this text: We focus on the question of how to research TCM as well as the question of the relation of Occidental and Chinese science. In this chapter we want to present the central ideas to answer these questions and to solve those scientific problems. Those ideas are developed by the concepts of the position of Constructive Realism. At first we want to give you an impression of what this theoretical proposal is like, while we are going to give reasons for this in the next chapter.

To summarise the ideas of Constructive Realism and to presents its concept for researching: To do a TCM adequate research we suggest to consider that there are differences between Western science and Chinese science respectively between their medical systems; to express the own and typical way of thinking of TCM – all together: to help the scientists to become aware of the special way of thinking and to understand their science.

If we consider this summary we find three central ideas: first the idea to consider the differences between the two sciences, second to express their typical way of thinking and third to be aware and to understand the peculiarity of their thinking. But what do they mean? – Those three ideas (that will be very important for our further arguing) suppose that TCM has its own approach to human body, health and illness, as well as an own way of constructing and structuring its medical system – that TCM can be understood as an own medical and scientific system. That means that TCM should be considered as one way of constructing a medical system to deal with health and illness of human being – one possible way besides others. This also means that TCM can coexist next to Western medicine as well as Western medicine next to TCM. Each of them has certain legitimacy, both may claim truth for their concepts and both may be incompatible to each other without doubting their legitimacy or their claim for truth. Based on the theoretical ideas of Constructive Realism and its concept of science as well as its application on TCM we can state that both systems are not compatible to each other and may not be blended because they are each based on different presuppositions of how to construct a scientific system.

Besides this essential idea to consider and to reflect the differences of the two sciences we suggest to focus on the typical way of thinking of TCM. To fulfill this we propose to emphasize on researching the original texts of TCM – in a special way. That means that considering the original texts does not only mean to try to translate those into modern language and modern categories of scientific thinking. Instead you should understand the original meaning by taking care of the original contexts and the presuppositions that were founding those documents. With this you would fulfill the named objective to acknowledge the typical and special way of thinking of TCM while considering its difference to Western Medicine. Because then you assume that TCM is based on certain central presuppositions that can be alternative and not common to those of another medical system respectively the Western type of medicine.

2.2 Theoretical reasoning: The position of "Constructive Realism"

Up to now we showed the way in that Constructive Realism answers the named questions. The next step is to explain how to come to such results and arguments. That means that in this chapter we are bound to state the theses and concepts of this position of philosophy of science founding this way of solving the scientific problem. In that sense we will explain (1) the main targets of Constructive Realism, (2) its ontology respectively its concept of the relation of science to its object, (3) its methodology to become aware of the special way of scientific thinking, and (4) its epistemology respectively its concept of knowledge in science and its specific problems.

2.2.1 The main targets of Constructive Realism: understanding in science

To understand the position of Constructive Realism as well as its concepts it is very useful to know about the problems it refers to. Because its objectives, strategies and concepts are to consider as a consciousness and reaction of certain problems that can be found in scientific work. And if you know about these problems you can understand the essential goals of Constructive Realism. This should help to understand its position and its concrete concepts that will be explained afterwards.

Constructive Realism deals with two certain problems of scientific work and one general problem in scientific thinking. These are 1) the problems of scientists and their questions they raise in the field of philosophy of science on the one hand and 2) the problem of knowledge in science on the other hand. 3) All together Constructive Realism refers to the general problem of scientific work: the problem of self-understanding respectively self-miss-understanding in science with all its consequences for work and results.

(1) The first problem Constructive Realism takes care of refers to the questions and problems scientists have in their scientific work. That means that Constructive Realism is no longer dealing with classic and typical questions of philosophy of science like the questions for the logical structure of science. Its target is not to answer the questions philosophers

of science raise – instead it focuses on the questions of scientists concerning their typical work. These questions concern worth and use of scientific results, but it is also at stake what their theses imply according to the world. Second there is the problem that it's often very difficult for scientists to translate their scientific knowledge in order to explain their results to people who are not trained in their field.

(2) The second specific problem of Constructive Realism is the problem about knowledge in science. To understand this problem in the way of Constructive Realism you have to differ between two certain ways of doing science: first the way of observing the rules of scientific systems and second the way of understanding of what is done with a scientific system. The second problem refers to the current tendency that science – especially natural sciences and sciences that have a specific affinity to the way of thinking of natural sciences –emphasizes the first way of scientific work: observing the rules and the working of a scientific system. In that sense science is considered in respect to its technological side and its working. But the problem is that scientists then don't really understand what they are doing. That means that they are able to apply the rules of their sciences and disciplines in a correct way and to come to certain results – but they often don't understand what they do, what their results mean or what the object of their research was thought to be. And this is an essential problem of scientific work: scientists are able to observe scientific rules, but they don't understand them.[1]

(3) If we summarise the two special problems of scientific work Constructive Realism focuses on, we can name a general problem of scientific work considering the perspective of this position. An essential problem in science is the problem of self-understanding or self-miss-understanding of scientists. That means that scientists have problems to understand their own doing, their way of thinking, their objects, their rules and their results – although they observe the rules of their sciences and disciplines correctly and although they can be considered as real and authentic scientists. To avoid miss-interpretations: Qualification respectively being professional on the one hand and self-understanding on the other hand do not form an opposition.

---

1   This issue will be discussed and explained more detailed in chapter 2.2.3.

Considering these problems – the scientists' consciousness of the worth of their results, the problems of translating one's system, the problem of the ability to observe the rules of a scientific system while not understanding them – we now can show you the essential targets of Constructive Realism: It wants to help the scientists to get to know about their thinking, to help them to make themselves comprehensible, to be able to understand what they are doing when they succeed in observing their scientific rules. It is its aim to give an impulse to scientists to reflect themselves, to support self-understanding in scientific work and to avoid self-miss-understanding and – as a consequence – defective developments in science. In this sense Constructive Realism can be considered as an authority respectively an instance of service for science[1].

2.2.2 Ontology of Constructive Realism: considering the differences

Let us return to the leading question of this article: We are questioning how to research TCM in an adequate way by considering the relation of TCM and Western science. Based on the concepts and arguments of Constructive Realism we would answer this question (as it was shown before) that we have to consider TCM as an own approach to human body, a special and legitimated way of constructing a medical system; that it has its own right to claim for truth and the status of science without contradicting the Occidental way of medicine respectively the one of Western school medicine; that TCM and Western medicine have to be considered as different and incompatible ways of constructing science.

But now the question occurs: How to come to such results? Respectively what concepts have we to use and what theses have we to assume in order to deduce this point of view? To answer this question we are going to take two steps: (1) We have to explain the ontological concept of Constructive Realism and its understanding of science and (2) we will apply this concept to TCM respectively the relation of Western and Chinese science.

(1) To avoid miss-interpretation of the following arguments we have to express the notion "ontology" as it is used here as well as the character of its

---

1   Wallner 1992a, p.199

concept: When we speak about the "ontology" of Constructive realism we consider it as the concept of the relation between science and its object. In this respect the ontology of Constructive Realism is not to consider as new metaphysics presenting new insights into the structure of the world. Instead this ontological concept focuses on the working of science. It is not the aim of the constructive realistic ontology to state what the world is like, instead it wants to explain how science works – this thought and delimitation is very important to consider in order not to get the following concept in a wrong way.

To explain the ontological concept of Constructive Realism and its understanding of the relation of science to its object we want to start with describing scientific work in general: In that respect let us consider two different levels in science, the level of language on the one hand and the level of the object on the other hand. On the first level, the linguistic level, science develops systems of propositions. These propositions are not to consider as descriptions of the objects they refer to, instead as rules of how to handle the amount of data of the object. That means that these propositions can be understood as instructions to control an amount of data of a certain field in science that tell us what we can expect when we do certain scientific actions. So, on this first level we find instructions of how to handle data, instructions that don't describe the objects.

On the second level, the level of data, we find the fundament of the first level. Because on this level we find data the propositions refers to. There we have to consider the important question of the character of these data. It is the question whether they really are to consider as absolute objective data unspoiled by subjectivity? – Based on the results of modern research on philosophy of science we have to reject this attitude and instead to confess that these data are no "purely data" and no "purely objective data". Instead the data, the propositional system refers to, are to consider as a result of an approach that is lead by theory. That means that every so called "data" is the result of a selection and an exclusion of certain qualities of the object science refers to; that scientists focus on certain aspects of the analyzed object being guided by certain targets, questions, respects, (in many cases) by technological possibilities and some implicit theoretical convictions. – So we have to confess that the basis of science is the process of selecting and excluding certain aspects of the analyzed object, a process that is guided by theory.

This insight into the basis of science is the point where Constructive Realism is developing its ontological concept respectively its understanding of the relation of science and its object. Considering the named insight Constructive Realism states that science can be understood as artificial and constructed systems of data and propositions; that science is to consider as a constructed "microworld", a world that selects and reduces qualities in certain respects and that is important for our thinking and our actions as well.

In that sense we can differ between two essential und fundamental dimensions of scientific work: "Realität" and "Wirklichkeit". These notions are words of German language. We seriously insist to use the German words and not to translate them because both mean "reality" in English what blurs this essential differentiation. So we are going to use the German words to express the difference and different dimensions of scientific work.

But what does this difference mean? What does it refer to? As mentioned the notions "Realität" and "Wirklichkeit" name two different dimensions in science. "Realität" describes the scientific microworlds, the world that is constructed by the selection and exclusion of qualities of the object, a process that is guided by theory. On the other hand "Wirklichkeit" describes the genuine world, the world that depicts the fundament for Realität and the basis for the selection and reduction. This is the world that we are living with and that keeps us alive (for example when it feeds us).

After the characterization of the two worlds established by Constructive Realism, we have to focus on the relation of those worlds and ask the question whether and in what way they are connected: As it was already mentioned those "microworlds" or "Realitäten" in general are to consider as artificial worlds, as results of scientific actions. Concerning the relation of Realität to Wirklichkeit we have to propose that in any case there is a reference of Realität to Wirklichkeit as far as the constructions are selecting and excluding the qualities of Wirklichkeit. Thus we have to name two characteristics of this relation: first the reference and second the reduction of the manifoldness of Wirklichkeit. This also means that we have to reject the idea that the scientific systems and their data systems were identical to Wirklichkeit respectively that Wirklichkeit was structured in the same way as the scientific systems. Thus as a consequence we have to concede that in respect to thinking we do not describe the scientific objects or the world and second in respect to acting we replace Wirklichkeit by Realität that is reduced on the one hand but still working on the other hand.

To illustrate this thesis of replacing nature with an example: Take the problem of heart diseases. To react on such heart problems science – especially Western medicine – developed and constructed an own data system and with that an own microworld to handle those problems. By certain surgeries medicine replaces the deficient natural organ by an artificial organ. One the one hand this can be very effective actually while on the other hand it just replaces some aspects of nature but not all. That means that some nature always remains around this microworld what sometimes may evoke new and not predicted problems.

To summarise the theoretical conclusions Constructive Realism draws out of the idea that science is a process of selection and exclusion of qualities guided by theory: The scientific systems are to consider as an artificial and constructed microworld that is based on selecting, excluding and reducing a world we name "Wirklichkeit". But this reduction does not reject that there is a reference of Realität to Wirklichkeit. So we can propose the relation of Realität and Wirklichkeit in general as a relation of reference and reduction or as a reductive reference. – With that we now can name the character of the scientific systems as constructions that have a reductive reference to their objects and world they analyze. But we also can dismiss the possible objection that scientific systems were to consider as illusionary and fictive.

(2) Let us apply these arguments on the relation of Western and Chinese science: Based on the insights of Constructive Realism we can consider science the way that it is not in correspondence with nature while science is a job that constructs models which are connected with nature in a specific way. In the last 50 years the main point of the research on the structure of Western science is that science is a manifoldness of constructions of our reference to the world. We have many different constructions of these references. Some of them are compatible, some of them are incompatible. Therefore there is one thing you should consider: There is mani-

foldness of perceiving the world, not just one way and not just one solution – as the Western science usually believes.

In the last 15 years we have seen another aspect which was so hard to understand for European scientists especially for European Philosophers of science: that science also is dependent from culture. That means that science is guided by cultural convictions. Therefore it is fair to contend that we have a Western science or European science. This is a term we use in difference to a Chinese science, in difference to sciences or scientific attempts of other cultures. It is fair because in this case we contend that there is not only one way to make a structure of the world and that there are different ways to form those structures of the world in an intellectual manner.

To summarise these thoughts and to refer them to the leading question concerning the research on TCM and the relation of Chinese and Western science: On the one hand we have the understanding of Constructive Realism of the nature of science – that science is to consider as an artificial construction that selects and reduces certain qualities of an originally world guided by theory so that it has a reductive reference to the world. On the other hand we have to concede that there are several and different possibilities of referring to the world, different ways of selecting and reducing. Based on this reductive reference and the legitimate manifoldness of different references we can propose that TCM and its system are as well to consider as a scientific system that has its own and alternative reference to the world and its own approach to its object. Thus it also has a legitimate claim for truth without getting into contradiction with other and different systems like the Western medicine. It also can be not compatible to Occidental school medicine as both have different ways of constructing their microworlds.[1]

2.2.3 Methodology of Strangification: expressing the peculiarities

Now let remind us of the proposal of Constructive Realism to answer the leading questions of our thinking: Based on its concepts and ideas it was

---

1   We will focus this aspect of *incompatibility* in chapter 2.3 more detailed.

suggested first to consider the differences and peculiarity of the two sciences of Western and traditional Chinese medicine and second to express the typical way of the thinking of TCM. – By explaining the ontology of Constructive Realism we already emphasized the first suggested advice to consider the differences. Based on this we now can focus on the second advice to express the peculiar way of the thinking of TCM. That means that we have to stress the question of how to manage to express the way of thinking? What shall we do to get to know in what way a scientific Realität is constructed? How can we understand what qualities are selected and what are excluded? How can we achieve to know what are the fundamental presuppositions of constructing a scientific system? – To answer these questions and to fulfill the named objective to express the typical way of thinking of TCM we will take two steps: (1) we are going to explain the theoretical concept and procedure of the methodology of Constructive Realism while (2) we want to combine its concept and our objective to express the way of thinking of TCM.

(1) The methodology of Constructive Realism is called "strangification" in English. "Strangification" is an artificial word, a translation of the German word "Verfremdung". This methodology comes from the field of hermeneutics. Hermeneutic is a way of interpreting and understanding. This methodology is to consider as the strategy of Constructive Realism to solve the problems of science respectively philosophy of science that it tries to deal with as well as to fulfill its main objectives. To understand its concepts you have to know two central ideas: first the theoretical targets of the methodology and second its procedure. To explain them:

The method has a number of essential objectives that lead its procedure. You can find those objectives in many ideas and concepts of Constructive Realism that were already mentioned and explained as well as you can deduce them from the central problems Constructive Realism is dealing with. The method tries to stimulate and to support self-understanding of scientists that means to let them understand what they are doing in their scientific work and what their results and insights really mean. It tries to improve the scientific understanding by expressing and mentioning the implicit theoretical presuppositions that are founding the scientific theories, arguments, approaches, conclusions and results; by making the way of constructing Realität explicit as well as the character of the reductive reference to the world. By showing up the implicit fundaments of scientific thinking this method tries to fulfill the aim to support self-understanding in science and to save the scientific claim for knowledge[1].

Considering the last arguments we now have shown you the essential goals of the methodology of Constructive Realism. But how can we manage to do this? How do we have to proceed to support self-understanding, to save the claim for knowledge and to express the implicit fundaments of scientific thinking? – To fulfill these named goals the methodology follows a simple strategy: Take a scientific system or concept out of its original context and put it into another and different context. The more different this other context is the better for the use of this methodology.

To explain this we will need a preliminary remark: Strangification is based on the concept that science or disciplines are systems of propositions that are based on certain presupposition. These presuppositions have the meaning that they depict the condition for the truth of a proposition. That means that every proposition or every medical advice is just true under certain conditions. This also means that we cannot say that a scientific proposition is true under all conditions. So if we want to find out the true content of a proposition, a concept or a medical advice, we have to consider its presupposition. And here you can find the aim of this methodology: It is to show and to raise the conditions or the presuppositions that are necessary for the truth of a proposition, a concept, a term or a medical advice. But how can we manage that? Strangification goes the following way to get to know those presuppositions: We take the system of propositions, the terms or advices out of their original context and put it in a different context – and as said, the more different it is the better for the research.

What happens if we mix scientific systems of propositions with different contexts? As a consequence of this procedure some aspects of the scientific concepts are getting absurd and don't make any sense because they are missing certain presupposition that are needed for their truth and

---

1   also see chapter 2.2.4

that are not given in the different context. At this point you can see what presupposition you have to have to get a true and a not-absurd sentence. So this absurdness is the point where you have to emphasize research. Because this proceeding enables you to get to know what implicit and not reflected fundaments a scientific system or concept is built up upon without being reflected.[1] So by using this method of strangification, by changing the contexts of the scientific systems or concepts you can become aware of the implicit presuppositions that are needed to have a true and a meaningful scientific system or concept.

To illustrate this mentioned procedure with an example of our field of research: As one example we want to refer to the scientist Kaptchuk: It is about the diseases of the stomach. In the Western world we have the diseases of the stomach which are leading to surgery and so on. In Chinese medicine diseases of the stomach have six situated functions of the body. It is a different way of understanding. It has six different solutions just for the one solution of the Western world. Therefore if you take the methodology of strangification for this problem of the diseases of the stomach you can become aware of the presupposed fundament for the different medical concepts. Further examples would be the concept of blood pressure or the five elements.

To summarise the methodological concept: The application of the method of strangification proceeds by taking a scientific system or concept into a context respectively a field that is very untypical for the use of the scientific system. Because of this unusual mixing theoretical senselessness and absurdity will occur expressing what ideas have to be presupposed so that a concept or an argument becomes true and meaningful. By achieving insights into the implicit and mostly not reflected theoretical basis the scientists are able to become aware of the way they are constructing Realität while doing their scientific work and what their reference to the world is like.

(2) Before we were showing and explaining the methodological concept of strangification theoretically. Now we want to apply it on the research of TCM and on the leading question of our argumentation to fulfill the idea to

---

1   Greiner 2006, p.44

express the typical way of thinking of TCM. The following arguments are more to consider as a description of a concept of research and less as concrete results. To do an effective and meaningful research on TCM by considering and expressing its own way of thinking we give you the following advice: Go back to the original text and study them in a certain way!

This is important for contemporary Chinese researchers or medical doctors as well as for Western scientists. It is not a question of translating the text instead it is a question of understanding it in a context which was adequate to the original context. We now could object that we can not constitute the Chinese world two thousand years ago. So what shall we do in this situation? First rule is we must not translate literally because the word in the new context, even the Chinese word, has another context and therefore another theoretical fundament than the same word in the old text. Thus translation won't be able to help. Instead we have to do one thing: We have to take a look at the context of the concepts. It is the context of medical advices we suggest to focus on. This is the point where you have to apply and to use the named methodology of strangification: To reconstruct the original context and to express the necessary theoretical fundament that depicts the condition for truth and meaning of those texts you should use strangification. Another example for this procedure was to compare the Chinese meridians with the Western nerve system. So by the use of this methodology you should become aware of the essential basis of TCM while it should help you to understand your own discipline and your own science better.

2.2.4 Epistemology of Constructive Realism: working and understanding

At this point we want to remind ourselves of the steps we already took to answer the leading questions. To do a TCM adequate research we propose to consider the two sciences as different ways of doing science (ontological concept) on the one hand while expressing the own and special way of thinking of them by using a certain procedure (methodological concept) on the other hand. Now let us stress the last of the three ideas of Constructive Realism to answer the leading questions that were named in chapter 2.1. This third aspect of our answer focuses on the understanding of scientists of their sciences and disciplines. It is already implied in the first two aspects but we now want to discuss it explicitly as it deals with an important problem of researching TCM and Western school medicine on the one hand and a central scientific problem in the present on the other hand.

It concerns the modality that means the manner of doing science respectively researching TCM. It deals with the question whether scientists just apply scientific rules correctly or whether they understand what they are doing; whether science is done in a technological respectively functional respect or whether science claims to offer insights and knowledge. This is an important differentiation we have to consider to improve the research on TCM: technology and knowledge respectively functioning and understanding. To support an understanding of this scientific problem we have to explain the epistemological concept of Constructive Realism as well as its advice how to deal with this problem.

The epistemological concept of Constructive Realism focuses on the worth and character of the scientific results respectively the mentioned two different ways of doing science – observing and understanding. It deals with the problem of "instrumentalism" that means the wide spread tendency in science especially in natural sciences and those sciences that have an affinity to them. It is the tendency to identify science with technology and the aspect of working, functioning and regulating world. Then science is always related to claims like improving the conditions and standards of every day life and work.

But what is the problem if science is done in that way? The problem of this proceeding is that science then is reduced to observing rules, functioning and controlling world what is not equivalent to understanding and knowledge. So if there is an emphasis on this technological side of science it is problematic for science to claim for knowledge. On the other hand this focus on functioning supports the reduction and loss of possibilities of reflecting and deciding in science.

If we say that functioning and knowledge can not be identified and that a difference between them has to be considered we have to answer the question about the concept of knowledge and its difference to working. So let us name and reflect our understanding of "knowledge". – Knowledge does not mean to succeed in scientific working by observing scientific rules in a correct manner or to have a scientific concept function. Knowledge doesn't also mean to know about the object of a certain science or discipline. Instead it means to know about the way of constructing and structuring an object. It is to know about those aspects that are implicitly focused and excluded from the object of science when it produces and presents its theories. That means that knowledge always means to go beyond a scientific system, its rules and functioning. It is the objective of this proceeding to express the implicit presuppositions that depict the fundament of the functioning processes. So it is to show on what theoretical concepts those processes are based on. – But let us ask: What is the advantage of knowledge in scientific work? The answer reads: Knowledge in relation to functioning opens and broadens the possibilities of scientific thinking and acting while it reduces misunderstanding and defective developments in scientific concepts.

Let us refer this differentiation between functioning and knowing to our question and our focus on researching TCM. If we consider this difference in the way of doing science we can express and refine the manner of this research. When we are researching TCM it should not be our general objective just to know the medical rules and the advices this medicine gives, to know how to apply them to cure a sick person and how to observe its rules. Instead of focusing this respect of correct use and working we should stress on the way of understanding and knowledge respectively on such kind of research. That means we should emphasize on understanding the rules, their concepts and their way of thinking respectively the way they construct their object, what respects of the body they focus and what they exclude. Then we can do a more effective and more error resistant research on TCM because we know about the implicit presuppositions respectively the theoretical fundament. This knowledge will help us then to avoid misunderstanding and problematic use of this medical system. For example if we know about the way of thinking and constructing of the system of TCM and know about its genuine and peculiar theoretical basis we would not try to mix TCM and Western medicine respectively their concepts so easily. Then we also would not combine concepts of those two medicines to develop new ways of healing. In that sense we can say that we may not blend Chinese herbs and Western medicine in the field of pharmacology for example.

So we get more resistant against problematic scientific decisions and then we can avoid lots of decisive and expensive errors in the work of science and the realisation of scientific results. Thus the manner of researching TCM should not just emphasize on a correct use of its procedures instead it should explicitly focus on understanding to become more competent and effective.

At this point we can name another aspect of the use of the methodology of strangification respectively another advantage of its research. The use of this method and its proceeding as it was described and explained in chapter 2.2.3 also supports this way of doing science by understanding and knowledge. That means that by the use of strangification you achieve the possibilities to go beyond a scientific system and to express its fundaments and finally to understand it.

2.3 Application: considering, expressing and understanding the differences

Before we want to do another step let us review our argumentation: We focus on the question of an effective and adequate research on TCM while we are explicitly taking care of the relation of TCM and Western science. To answer this question we were proposing a concept of a certain way of researching TCM by considering the ideas and theories of the philosophical position of Constructive Realism: First it is to take into consideration that TCM and Western medicine are to understand as different and special ways of doing science. Second it is to research on expressing this genuine way of thinking. Third it is to do a research in the manner and the objective of understanding instead of functioning. We gave reasons for those three traits with central concepts of the named position of Constructive Realism: its ontology, its methodology and its epistemology.

With those ideas and theories we were developing a concept of researching TCM. Now as the next step we finally want to apply this concept and carry it out. So in this chapter we are now going to present some insights into the special way of the thinking of TCM and Western science applying the ideas we have explained before. To do this we want to focus on two aspects: 1) we want to show essential differences between Occidental and Chinese Medicine that will explain their incompatibility; 2) we want to name mistakes that can happen if you research TCM as well as we want to mention some advices that should help you to improve this scientific work.

(1) At first we want to present some essential differences in the way of thinking of Western and Occidental science. These are important to consider and to understand if you want to research TCM. – The first aspect to mention is the concept of experience. The Chinese way is a different way as the Western one. You can say that Chinese science has a big experience but this is not the same as the experience of the way of Western science. It is not to decide which type of experience is the better one. These are two different ways to experience the world.

The Western way of experience is the following: you must take out the subject, you must go back from nature and take out all what is human related. You must make nature completely objective, this means you must reduce your subjectivity to zero. This is clearly impossible but it was always the intention of all scientists in the Western world that subjectivity must be taken out. Otherwise your results do not have a scientific value, is not scientific.

In the Chinese way experience is not guided by this idea that subjectivity is to be taken out. It takes another direction: instead subjectivity is taken in. You are always referring to the master who offers these experiences. –Therefore if you speak about evidence based science, be careful: For Chinese science this has a different meaning than for the Western science.

A second different point is the question of generality, generality in scientific work: You know in the Western science generality has a high value. The more general a theory, the more specific is its worth. And therefore the Western world, the Western languages have this concept of the universals, of the most general concepts which are covering all. In Chinese language the way is another one what means that the way of generalising is usually not done. Let's say they go the sideway. The wood is a sum of trees, is not a specific concept for instance.

If you study Chinese science, you always have to be aware that universality has no big importance for them. Very important are – let's introduce this term – "intermobiles". Because what they are doing is not based on abstraction to more general terms, they go a sideway and connect other aspects with the first one. This is a different way of making experience: to connect other qualities and other objects with an object to understand this object better.

In the Western way you must take out some qualities from the object to get a scientific result. Therefore the scientific result in the Western world always is reducing qualities. Therefore it is always a big decision which qualities are important and which qualities are not.

A main point of Chinese understanding of the world is the relation of body and mind. So many Philosophers since Plato are thinking about this question of how the relation of body and mind can be thought in an adequate and in a true way. And as you know as medical doctors this is very important for medicine, for medical doing. But this is a typical Western question.

In the Chinese way you don't have the body-mind-problem. If they speak about mental problems, they do it by words connected with the body. In the beginning there is no difference like in the Western world and this causes/ a lot of consequences for science. Therefore psychology for instance is a new science for China because it is a typical Western science. To set mind as an autonomous object is very untypical for Chinese science. But China today is not the old China, is not the China of the TCM – always be aware of this point.

Just a small other point – small but also important: The concept of nature. Even today and even among people who are not religious or something like this you can find the following implicit conviction: that the world has a beginning and that the world is something which is constructed, which has rules and so on. This was the basis of Western science from the beginning. This is a basis coming from Plato and Aristotle and is connected with Christian thinking. Therefore it is so strong over all the hundreds of years and therefore it is guiding a lot of science in the Western world. For instance take a look at cosmology: They ask about the beginning of the world. You can consider this question as a pseudo-problem. It is a typical culturally induced problem which is no question for Chinese thinking.

A very important difference is the problem of holism. A lot of scientists assume that the difference between Western and Chinese thinking is holistic. This does not tell anything and it is wrong too. There is also a holistic thinking in the Western world. But this is different from the holism in the Chinese world. The difference is: If in the Western world we are looking for holism, we are making a construction. We start with single experiences continuing to general experiences while we are mostly using inductions which are unknown in Traditional Chinese Medicine. Holism in Chinese thinking is the condition of thinking not the result of a way of reasoning.

(2) At last we want to mention some hints about mistakes and effective ways of researching TCM. Let us begin with popular errors: There are four basic makes that can occur and that should be avoided:

- A common mistake of Westerners is that they are looking for similarities. This is the wrong way from the beginning.
- Another mistake is the attempt to give TCM-propositions a scientific legitimation. If you understood the arguments before, you know that this is wrong. It is impossible to find a legitimation for TCM that is coming from Western science. This is similar to find a legitimation for love by bio-chemistry. This is simply not adequate as you understand.
- A third mistake is to take out TCM-advices out of their original contexts. This is the usual way of the Western world because usually we do not know the texts. We just know small parts of the text and based on these small parts we pick up some words that are interesting for us.
- Another mistake is to use terms that are loaded by Western science.

And at the end let us mention some advices what you should observe if you research TCM:

- First replace theory by network! If you research on TCM do not ask for theory at first, ask for the network.
- Look at differences and not at similarities! Do not generalise!
- Look for examples instead of explanations!
- Try to reduce your position to an observer!

3. Summary: answering the leading questions

In the last part of this text we finally want to come back to the fundament of our argumentation respectively the questions that were leading our thinking. So let us remind us of these central questions and the concepts we mentioned and explained to answer the questions so that we finally are able to give concrete answers for the questions and problems of the research on TCM.

The problem and the question concerning the research on TCM we are dealing with consists of two parts: there are two central questions that are connected with each other and that are both to answer if we want to improve the research on TCM. On the one hand we have the question how to improve the research on TCM by being effective and having a correct approach. This first question leads us to the second question as we have to ask in what way we have to approach to TCM. This second questions is motivated by the contemporary scientific discussion between modern Occidental medicine and science on the one hand and traditional Chinese medicine and its science on the other hand. The second question focuses on this relation and wants to clarify what this relation of the two sciences is like. Thus altogether we are reflecting the question in what way we have to approach to TCM to have a correct and insofar effective research on TCM and its typical way of thinking and healing.

Now let us mention the essence of our way to answer these leading questions respectively the named scientific problem. In that respect we have to mention two aspects, 1) the character of our answer and 2) the methodological concept of a TCM research.

(1) If you want to name the main character of our answer you have to consider that our concept of answering this question is to understand as pre-considerations for a TCM research that reflects the approach to TCM. That means that our concept has to be understood as a methodological reflection. Our approach to this problem is founded by theories and concepts of philosophy of science that we were applying to the research on TCM and the relation of its system and the system of Western medicine.

(2) In this sense of developing preceding methodological reflections by applying ideas of the field of philosophy of science we were preparing a certain methodological concept of researching TCM. This concept consists

of three parts: first it is to consider that there are fundamental differences between the scientific and medical system of the traditional Chinese thinking and the one of the modern Occidental one. Thus we secondly propose to express the own and special way of thinking of TCM and Western science in order to consider the differences of the two sciences. As well as we thirdly characterise this research on TCM as a modality of understanding instead of having the systems and their concepts function.

These aspects of a methodological concept of a research on TCM are deduced from the theoretical approach of Constructive Realism which is a modern position of philosophy of science that focuses on the competence of understanding science. The first trait of the named concept was argued with the understanding of Constructive Realism of science. In that way science is considered as an artificial construction that has a reductive reference to the world and its object by selecting and excluding qualities of the focused object of one science. As far as many and different ways of a selective reference to the world are possible we can concede that TCM has an alternative way of thinking next to the Occidental way of thinking without doubting the scientific status of any of those sciences [1]. – In order to get to know the differences between the named sciences respectively to achieve insights into the special way of thinking of TCM; and in order to fulfill the second trait of our suggested concept of expressing the peculiarity of TCM we presented and explained the methodology of Constructive Realism named "strangification". It proceeds by mixing scientific systems of propositions with untypical contexts or fields of application with the effect that the occurring absurdities show up the implicit presuppositions that are founding the scientific construction as well as its claims for truth[2]. – The third strait of understanding TCM instead of having it function was argued with the concept of Constructive Realism about the fundamental differentiation in scientific work: working and knowledge. In order to have a research that is resistant against methodological and theoretical errors and mistaken scientific developments or problematic realizations of results of science we advised to focus on the way of understanding instead of functioning[3]. – This concept of an adequate way of a research on TCM is

---

1   see 2.2.2
2   see 2.2.3
3   see 2.2.4

complemented by a number of concrete insights into essential presuppositions of traditional Chinese and Occidental science. In that respect we were mentioning their different understandings of experience, generality, the relation of body and mind, of nature and holism[1].

That means altogether we were focusing on the questions in what way we have to approach to TCM to have an adequate research. We answered this question to research TCM in the way of considering a fundamental scientific difference between TCM and Western medicine explicitly, of expressing their own and peculiar ways of thinking while focusing on understanding the medical systems instead of having them function. With that we should have a good and fertile (methodological) fundament to do an adequate that means a correct and effective research on its way of thinking and healing.

Reference

Greiner, Kurt u.a. 2005, Verfremdung – Strangification. Multidisziplinäre Beispiele der Anwendung und Fruchtbarkeit einer epistemologischen Methode, Frankfurt/Main: Peter Lang.

Kaptchuk, Ted J. 2006, Das große Buch der chinesischen Medizin. Die Medizin von Yin und Yang in Theorie und Praxis, Frankfurt/ Main: Fischer.

Wallner, Fritz 1992a, Konstruktion der Realität. Von Wittgenstein zum Konstruktiven Realismus, Wien: Universitätsverlag.

Wallner, Fritz 1992b, Acht Vorlesungen über den Konstruktiven Realismus, Wien: Universitätsverlag.

Wallner, Fritz 2002, Die Verwandlung der Wissenschaft. Vorlesungen zur Jahrtausendwende, ed. v. Martin J. Jandl. Hamburg: Kovac.

Wallner, Fritz 2006a, Traditionelle Chinesische Medizin. Eine alternative Denkweise, Aitrang: Windpferd.

Wallner, Fritz 2006b, What Practitioners of TCM should know. A Philosophical Introduction for medical doctors, Frankfurt/Main: Peter Lang.

Wallner Fritz 2006/7, What Practitioners of TCM should know. A Philosophical Introduction for medical doctors. [Translated into Chinese], Peking: Higher Education Press 2006. Announced for 2007.

---

1   see 2.3

Zhang Qicheng

The Cultural Characteristics of Chinese Medical Terminology and its Comparative Analysis in the Context of Western Medicine

Translated by Lena Springer

Traditional Chinese medical studies are a kind of medicine which is based on Chinese traditional culture, and which has rich cultural connotations. The theoretical system of Chinese medicine has taken shape through its application (lit. in its function) within the concepts and way of thought of Chinese traditional culture. It differs from Western medicine and modern scientific terminology; it contains a lot of terminology from Chinese philosophy actually. Not explaining it on the background of traditional culture but just starting the explanation of several definitions from concepts is far too less an effort. What's more, the definitions in text books and reference books, in many cases, still require further discussion. Therefore, one must start with the cultural origin of these concepts and terminology to truly capture the conceptual terms of Chinese medicine as well as the connotations and nature of the theories.

If Chinese medicine is internationalised and modernised nowadays, firstly, the standardisation problem of the translation of the Chinese medical terminology has to be solved. The translations of the expressions and the terminology of Chinese medicine – no matter whether by experts from China or by distinguished overseas experts – are not unified. Some translations make one cry and laugh greatly. For example, "wuzang liufu" has been translated as "five storehouses and six palasts", "baihu lijie" (pain in the joints due to swelling) has been translated as "the white tiger is jumping", "gongsun" (the name of an acumoxa point) has been translated as "grandfather and grandson". Can one imagine how such translation could ever spread Chinese medicine accurately?

As for the translation of the [traditional] Chinese medical names and terminology, while respecting the rules of English translation, the problem of the difference between Chinese and Western culture is of even more importance, only thus can the English language in its dynamic but authentic shape express the deep meaning(s) of Chinese traditional culture which the terminology connotes. In cases when correct and suitable direct translation is not possible in English, the ultimate principle ought to be the cultural connotations of Chinese medicine itself. The reason is that, naturally, the problem of the English translation of Chinese medicine reflects the difference between Chinese and Western culture (including the way of thought and the expression of logic). In no way can this difference be blurred for the sake of the convenience of the Westerners' comprehension process.

Below, I state the most fundamental terminology and categories of Chinese medical studies – qi, yinyang, wuxing – as examples, and discuss the cultural characteristics of the Chinese medical terminology and its way of thought.

Qi

"Qi" is the Chinese pinyin of 气, it has already become the common English (way of) translation, this is the particularity of the concept "qi". Even though the translation problem is solved, its definition has caused problems. "The Great Chinese TCM dictionary" explains it as follows: (1) refined nutritive substance flowing within the body; (2) generally denoting the function of the internal organs and tissues; (3) one of the affected phases or stages in acute febrile disease (wenbing bianzheng). Some text books name qi "the energy of life". "Qi" is one of the fundamental concepts of Chinese thought. The manifestation of any invisible force is called qi. All the above mentioned definitions are not complete enough. If only these definitions are introduced, the students – especially foreign students – have no means to grasp the connotations of qi correctly; moreover, the relation between the different meanings of qi can hardly be clarified. Therefore, the explanations have to start from the cultural background.

"Qi" originally is an important category of the main Chinese philosophy. It has been used by a number of philosophers to account for the origin of the universe, and the world. "Qi" already appears on the inscriptions on bones or tortoise shells of the Shang dynasty (ca. 16th BC-11th BC), and it originally denotes an existing substance of bodily condition, as in "yunqi" (literally cloud-qi), vapour, smoke and fog, wind etc. The concept "qi" is mentioned first in classical documents as an explanation of earth quakes in "guoyu zhouyu" (780 AD, the end of the Western Zhou Dynasty) by Bo Yanfu. During the Spring and Autumn period (770-476 BC), both Laozi and Konfuzius wrote about "qi". In the period of the Warring States (476-221 BC), *Guanzi, Mengzi, Zhuangzi, Xunzi* all mention "qi", but mostly from a philosophical perspective. In the Han dynasty (206 BC-220 AD), "qi" had already become an important category that explains the cosmos in itself/ as a noumenon, continuing the theory of the *Guanzi* about "jingqi" [essentielles Qi according to Unschuld] the school of thought "yuanqi" [the ancestors' qi or pectoral qi according to Unschuld] came up.

If we look at the alterations of the connotations of "qi", they changed from having a form to not having a form, from material to abstract. That is, it changed from air, gas of the natural world to all the entire formless re- fined substance, [its meaning] extended from high-quality (jingliang) maize (as in the unsimplified character 氣) to the essence of all things (as in "jingqi"), from the concrete material that all things in the univers are built from to the fundamental factor of life in the universe that transcends form, the mutual link between heaven, earth, sensed by all things. "Qi" as a phi- losophical category has, among others, the characteristics: transcending form (metaphysical), dynamic, linking, basic.

Chinese medical studies has lent the philosophical category "qi", "qi" has achieved very broad usage in Chinese medical studies. In the *Inner Canon of the Yellow Emperor* (*Huangdi Neijing*), it is used as often as some three thousand times, moreover, the meaning of "qi" changed in a very complex way. However, its judgement and explanation requires just grasping the cultural background of this change of the concept "qi". Gen- erally speaking, "qi" as used in Chinese medical studies is a concept which explains the phenomena of the life of the human body. It both be- wares the basic connotations and characteristics of the philosophical category "qi", and it has its own particular connotations. The nature and movement of the human body, and the generation activity rules of the life of the human bodily, both are regarded as "qi" or the generating and changing process of "qi" according to Chinese medicine. "Qi" is used in Chinese medicine to explain the physical functions, the structure, and the pathological conversions of the human body. "Qi" is generally the refined substance of life as well as the functions of life, but, in any case, it is wrong to separate the two. According to investigation of the philosophical culture, Chinese traditional though tends not to separate ti and yong (ti-yong bufen), the base and the application, the capacity and the action, the organism and the function, substantial "qi" and functional "qi" are not separable, substantial "qi" manifests itself as functional "qi", functional "qi" depends on substantial "qi". The *Great Chinese-English Medical Dictionary* just as the common text books (including the Chinese medicine text books) usually do not elucidate this relation. The fundamental reason for this is that the Chinese cultural background knowledge is ignored.

Yinyang

The definition according to the *Great Chinese-English Medical Dictionary* is "a general term for two opposite aspects of matters in nature, which are interrelated with each other". "yin" and "yang" are not explained concretely, but only "yang-qi" and "yin-qi" are explained. Yin-qi: "one aspect of the two opposites, as compared with yang-qi which denotes functional activity while yin-qi denotes substance." "yang-qi" is explained just as the opposite of "yin-qi". Some expert text books in English explain "yinyang" as "the principle of opposite" which "divides every phenomenon into its two contrary components". Both explanations deserve discussion. Combining the cultural background and the formulation process of the "yinyang" theory allow for clarifying its connotations.

The origin of the "yinyang" concept originates in prehistoric times. In the beginning, "yin" and "yang" meant a shady and a sunny place respectively. From the *yijing* which was written during the late Shang dynasty (1700-1100 BC) until the late Zhou dynasty (770-256 BC), the "yinyang" concept had ripened to a rather mature state. Up to the Western Zhou dynasty (1100-770 BC), the two characters "yinyang" had become a philosophical category already, used to explain all the natural things and phenomena. For example, the high-ranking minister of Zhou (1100-256 BC) Xuanwang, Guo Wengong, explained the unfreezing of the earth, spring thunder etc. with yinyang as two qi (yinyang erqi). In the late Spring and Autumn period (770-476 BC) Fan Li of the country Yue applied "yinyang" to the art of warfare; Laozi (Zhou dynasty, 6th century/604-531 BC) stated that "yinyang" exists in all things (wanwu fuyin er baoyang); in the period of the Warring States (476-221 BC), Zou Yan firstly integrated yinyang and wuxing to explain socio-historic changes.

Of course, "yinyang" thought has been systematized, theorized to an unprecedented state through the *yichuan*. The *yichuan* established the theoretical system of Chinese traditional "yinyang" thought and "yinyang" philosophy.

The *Inner Canon of the Yellow Emperor* (*Huangdi Neijing*) (206 BC-240 AD) made use of the "yinyang" philosophy and advanced "yinyang" to the metaphysical level of "dao". Plain questions, Great Analysis of the Yin-yang Phenomenon (Suwen yinyang yingxiang dalun): "Yinyang, the dao of heaven and earth, order and law of all things, the parents of change, the origin of becoming and death, the seat of spirit." This means that field and earth, above and below, male and female, right and left, water and fire each are another name for /synonyms of "yinyang". The *Inner Canon of the Yellow Emperor*, in a further step, applies the "yinyang" concept to phenomena of the life of the human body, and turns the viscera (zang and fu), the channels (jing and luo), qi and blood, the organs and the openings of the body such as nose, eye and ear (guan and qiao), form and structure, the space between the skin texture and the subcutaneous flesh (couli), vigour (essence and spirit) etc. into types of "yinyang" which belong to it. Moreover, "yinyang" is also used to illustrate pathological changes of the human body, its diagnosis and pattern differentiation, principles and methods of treatment.

Through the investigation of the cultural background, it is easy to see that definition of "yinyang" as a "principle of opposites" in the respective text books is not complete enough. The explanation of "yinyang" in reference books as "a general term for two opposite aspects of matters in nature, which are interrelated with each other" is also not complete enough. "yinyang" is not just "opposite" but also harmonious and unified, it comprises mutual transformation. "Yinyang" is not fully equal to "contradictory" or "positive and negative"; "yinyang" does not only signify the opposite types of different things, but also the two mutually opposed and mutually harmonious sides of the same thing. "Yinyang" comprises function, levels, mutual opposition, harmony, mutual transformation and other characteristics.

Wuxing

The English translation of the Chinese medical terminology of wuxing is one of the puzzles of translation Chinese medicine. Momentarily, the following main translations exist: (1) five elements and (2) five phases. It is necessary to understand the origin and the changing connotations of "wuxing" to translate the meaning of "wuxing" correctly. According to the research by the respective experts, "wuxing" originates in the later Shang dynasty (1700-1100 BC); it took shape in the Western Zhou dynasty when the five concepts water, fire, wood, metal/gold and earth appeared; it took a first step to its mature form in the Spring and Autumn period (770-476 BC), when the theory of mutual generation/ maintenance appeared; in a next step to its mature form in the period of the Warring States (476-221 BC) appeared the theory of the mutual generation of wuxing as well as the theory combing yinyang and wuxing; deified in the Han dynasty (206 BC-220 AD), wuxing became the holy unchangeable world view, methodology, and persisted until the end of the Qing dynasty (1644-1911).

So what does wuxing mean? It has been explained by the *shangshu hongfan*, *chunqiu yuanming bao*, *baihu tongyi*, *shuowen jiezi*, *yiming*, *guangya*, *wuxing dayi*, and by modern scholars from the Republic and People's Republic of China. Whereas these explanations are not equal, in summary, it mainly means "five materials" (wu cai) and "five natures" (wu xing):

1. the five types of basic material in the natural world of the universe wood, fire, earth, metal/gold, water
2. belonging to the five basic functions: to moisten or to lubricate (water), inflammation (fire), to bent and to straight (wood), chang/ to follow and to eliminate (metal/gold), and sowing and reaping (earth)

Whereas the first meaning of "wuxing" was "five materials" in sense of five material substances, once it became a model of thought, once it became an important philosophical category, and additionally used in the field of Chinese medicine and in all the other classical disciplines, it did neither mean five kinds of material nor five substances of form and structure anymore. Instead, it turned into a matter of fact that expresses relation and function. In Chinese traditional words, "wuxing" is not "qi" or "ti" anymore, but it is "qi" or "xiang". Wuxing expresses the reality of relation, the reality of function, neither a material substance nor a substance that would have a form. Wuxing signifies five types of a principle, the complex relation between five types of things. Wuxing boils the complex relation between things down to the relations: to generate and to decrease/ digest, 乘侮, to succeed and recover, to control and change.

Many scholars are convinced that "wuxing" (or "qi") is linking bond between material and function, for example Joseph Needham (1900-1995) explains: "Naming the character 'xing' element, we will always feel that it does not come up to the meaning. The origin of the character 'xing' […] has just the meaning 'movement'. Chen Mengjia for instance states that the five 'xing' are five very strong movements that never stop circulating, but that they are not a negative, unmoving basic (main) substance." Pang Pu holds the opinion that "xing" was just as easily comprehensible as the literary meaning of the noun and also of the verb to move, 行用, march forward; both the two views exist and each evolves their entirely new world view.

In my opinion, wuxing as a model has been employed by Chinese medicine in a wider sense, and it does not have the meaning of the noun "element" anymore, neither does it have the meaning of the verb "to move". Just as "qi", it is a model. It does not have the so-called double meaning of substance and function anymore. Transition from the material substance to the reality of relation and function is the fundamental speciality of "wuxing" and of "qi".

The characteristic of thought according to "qi-yinyang-wuxing"

The fundamental terminology of Chinese medicine has built its own theoretical system of physiology, pathology, diagnosis and medical treatment. "qi – yinyang – wuxing" are the most fundamental models of thought of Chinese medical science, they sufficiently constitute the way of thought of Chinese medical science. The terminology "qi-yinyang-wuxing" has the following characteristics.

Transcending form (metaphysical)

The three terms of the terminology "qi-yinyang-wuxing" are no substantial or material concepts, but they are a model of thought about the immaterial. For example, the character "qi" appears already in the inscriptions on bones or tortoise shells of the Shang dynasty (ca. 16th BC-11th BC) in its early meaning of an existing substance in the form of a vapour. "Qi" has two conditions: one is the condensed, material condition; qi separated into tiny condensed bits that can be seen and touched. The other is the condition when it is diffused in all directions and has no form; the scattered tiny bits of qi can neither be seen nor touched because of their continuous movement. In the Western Zhou dynasty qi already changed from a substance that can be felt into an immaterial abstract concept. The material qi was commonly named form ("xing"), and the former immaterial qi was now commonly named "qi". "qi" transcends form, it does not have a form, but it is the reason (lit. root) of form. "Yinyang" used to mean the places that the sunlight does (yang) or does not (yin) reach. Later it meant two mutually interrelated substances, like the sun and the moon, the sky and the earth, water and fire, blood and qi, (the two characters of the word) soul, male and female etc. Since the Western Zhou dynasty, "yinyang" meant two immaterial "qi", and started to have a philosophical meaning as something abstract without form. "Wuxing" in early times meant the "five materials", that is the five basic substances and materials wood, fire, earth, metal/gold, and water. Later the belonging to these five kinds of material already transcended the material condition. According to this model, the five "zang" of Chinese medicine are not the five anatomic, morphological organs liver, heart, spleen, lungs, and kidneys. But they are the combination of many organs that have the five functions; the "wuzang" (zang as in zangfu) constituted in this way are obviously in a condition that transcends form.

Functional form

"qi-yinyang-wuxing" serves as a model; it has changed from a material substance to a functional reality. Although the first meaning of the expressions "qi" "yinyang" and "wuxing" was a certain material substance, but it not only became a model of thinking but also a philosophical category, moreover – as it was widely used in Chinese medicine – it did not indicate a matter or substance in the condition of a form, but its meaning transcended the function and attribute of form and structure. For example in the pre-Qin philosophical classics and in the *Inner Canon of the Yellow Emperor*, the main function of "qi" is: it is the origin of everything in heaven and earth, the fundamental condition of life, the intermediate everything in heaven and earth interact through. The meaning of "yinyang" shifted from a single substance which either backs yin and faces yang to a couple of functional attributes which are mutually opposed and face each other: anything that fulfils the function to move something, to be pleasantly warm, to stimulate (/excite), to diffuse or disperse, or to raise belongs to yang; anything that fulfils the function to stablilize, to cool down, to inhibit, to condense or crystallise, or to lower belongs to yin. "wuxing" changed from five substantial elementary materials (五行) to five fundamental functional attributes (五性), they are to moisten (water), inflammation (fire), to bent and to straight (wood), change/to follow and to eliminate (metal/gold), sowing and reaping (earth), as stated firstly yin the "shangshu, Hong Fan". Later explanation of wuxing basically do not differ from this definition. The five functional attributes changed evolved into five types, that is the five priciples of categorisation wood, fire, earth, metal/gold, and water. "The Spring and Autumn annals (770-476 BC), the twelth period by Lü", the "Book of Rites" (Liji) etc. start to mention wuxing as a principle to categorise seasons, rites, zangxiang (the state of the zang-viscera; orbisiconography according to Manfred Porkert), temperament, a certain place and all other things. Consequently, the original meaning is most complex, and can hardlz be clarified simply by measuring things. The system of the five zang established in The Inner Canon of the Yellow Emperor is the result of the model of wuxing, this system epresses the functional system of the five categories of the life of the human body.

Relational form

"qi-yinyang-wuxing" expresses a relational reality, not a substantial reality. Belonging to the relational thought, its characteristic is that it attaches importance to the relation between one substance with the other, and the relation between one part within a substance to the other, these relations are given more priority than the form of matter and their internal structure. For example, "qi" means an intermediate that links all things and the parts within them. Qi fills in between all matter just as within every substance.

Only due to the function of qi all things respond to each other, intermingle with each other to become an entity and all things become a whole through the connectedness of their internal parts. "yinyang" is also a relation, the relations of "yinyang" are: being the root of each other, mutually moving, vanish, transmit and respond, mutually control, fight and disturb each other, change and succeed each other etc. Furthermore, "wuxing" is a model of relations, the main relations between the wuxing are: to generate and to diminish (to digest), 乘侮, to succeed and recover, to control and change, etc. The author of this paper is convinced that compared to the Western "for elements" (water, fire, earth, air) and to the Indian "four sizes" 四大 (earth, water, fire, wind) "wuxing" are superior, and have also been transmitted for a longer period of time. The basic reason for this is the characteristic relational characteristic of wuxing.

Holistic form

The model "qi-yinyang-wuxing" is holistic, it covers all information, and it is universal. If we take zangxiang (藏象) as an example, the holism of the five zang-organs (wuzang 五脏) manifests itself in two aspects: Firstly, they are one, secondly, man and heaven are one. Each zang-organ covers any other zang-organ, and also all the information of the whole human body. Thus, ancient theory states that the five zang-organs store (zang 藏) each other. The *Plain Questions* mentions about yinyang that 凡阳有五，五五二十五, in Ming dynasty (1368-1644) Zhang Jiebin suggested that "the five zang-organs each have the subtly of the wuxing", and "the five zang each simultaneously are the five qi", Zhou Qingzhai suggests that "each zang-organ also has the spleen and the stomach". In Qing dynasty (1644-1911) He Mengduan suggested that "each zang has the wuxing". This makes clear that every zang-organ contains the information of the five zang-organs. Moreover, every zangfu contains the information of the cosmos and nature; this reflects the ideas that heaven and man are mutually respondent and are one. The model "qi-yinyang-wuxing" is a universal model of thinking, anzting is applied to this model. There is no place where they do not exist, nor time without them. I will discuss them separately. If "qi" is large, nothing is outside it, if it is small nothing inside. It fills every place and time between all things in the cosmos. Zhuangzi, Zhi Bei You (知北游): There is one qi anywhere in the world under heaven" (通天下一

气耳). Qi not only generates everything, but due to it everything that is congested in the whole process of its generation and storage is linked and not disrupted. "yinyang" and "wuxing" are of the same kind as the corresponding five kinds of qi, heaven and earth as well as all things contain the qi of yinyang and the wuxing at the same time yinyang and wuxing function as a particular categorisation method that can be applied to everything in the world.

Opposite form

The model "qi-yinyang-wuxing" is a model of oppositions. "yinyang", for example face each other, they are not absolute. Concrete manifestations of this are: Firstly, "yinyang" have to change according to a standard. Yinyang are determined by a standard, and cannot be determined by a single aspect, without a comparative standard they cannot be determined. If the standard of comparison is different, than the judgement of yinyang differs, too. If, for example, the standard of water is zero, the level minus one is yin and the level plus one is yang. If the standard of water is ten, the level of one is yin and the level of 11 is yin. Secondly, yinyang change according to a relation. Yinyang are no substance, and no quality of a substance, but yinyang express, the relation between substances. For example, as for the relation among the group of male and female, male is yang, femail is yin; however, as for the relation among parents and children, the mother (female) is yang and the son (male) is yin. Thirdly, there is yin within yang and yang within yin. Because yin and yang can be distinguished in layers, there is again yinyang within yinyang. For example, daytime is yang, and the night is yin; the first half of the day is yang (yang within yang), and the second half is yin (yin within yang), the first half of the night is yang (yang within yin), and the second half is yin (yin within yin). "wuxing" all the same changes according to a comparative standard and relation, similarly there are phenomena of all "wuxing" contained in each "xing". The opposition of yinyang manifests itself in its dynamic. In its philosophical meaning, "qi" differs (lit. stands separate from) form ("xing"); the form is material and static, "qi" is immaterial/ has no form and is dynamic. "qi" has the characteristcs that it moves and does not stop, it changes constantly, it is unseparable. The movement of qi is named "qiji" (the mechanism/ vitality of qi); it generates all kinds of change. Thus the change and bringing into being of heaven and earth and all things is named qihua, the change of qi. The theory of qihua has developed the two phases of the essential qi and the original qi. Qi has no substantial form and can permeate and link inbetween all the substantial things. It can enter any place and time. At the same time, qi can absorbe all the parts of matter and it can build all kinds of qi, such as yang-qi, yin-qi, heaven-qi, earth-qi, wind-qi, the qi of clouds etc.

Temporal sequence

The model "qi-yinyang-wuxing" is a model that attaches more importance to temporal attributes that to spatial attributes. The movement and change of qi has temporal attributes. "wuxing" is often used to express the sequence and process of change of five kinds of substance. The *Shangshu, Hong Fan* lists 1st water, 2nd fire, 3rd wood, 4th metal/gold, 5th earth", later this was explained as the periods of the development of substances. Still, the sequence of the wuxing has not been defined, there are differend orders in different works, what's more, there are different orders in single works, as for example in *Guanzi* and in the *Inner Canon of the Yellow Emperor* etc. different orders of the wuxing reflect the different perspectives on the appearances in the cosmos and the different perspectives on the periods of the movements of matter. Even though most works do not clarify the order of "one two three four five", if we look at all the orders of wuxing, some use orders of mutual generation, some use orders of mutual digestion and some just are just a mixture. Wuxing is coordinate with social history and with the four seasons of the year, it is used to clarify their circular periods and the change between prospering and decline. The model of the five zang-organs has the characteristics of temporality and process. According to the spatial position of the wuxing, the five zang-organs are situated in space as follows: above the heart (fire), below the kidneys (water), left to the liver (wood), right to the lungs (metal/gold), in the centre of the spleen (earth). This spatial order obviously is not the order of the organs of human anatomic physiology. As a matter of fact, it is a temporal order. The *Inner Canon of the Yellow Emperor* has mentioned the expression "four seasons – five zang-organs – yinyang" (see the *Plain Questions* on the channels, *jingluo bielun*). Hui Ticao said once: "the five zang (藏) are not of blood or flesh, but they [are characterised by] the four seasons".

In fact, the functional system of the five zang-organs reflects the temporal phases of the diminishing and becoming yinyang in the four natural seasons.

Subjective form

The author of this paper has suggested in a number of his earlier articles that Chinese medical studies are a functional, algebraic, generating science that discusses models, Western/ biomedicine is a substantial, geometric, structural science that discusses prototypes. The "qi", the "yinyang", and the "wuxing" etc. concepts of Chinese medical studies are genuine concepts of the natural sciences, they also have a special connotation of the human sciences, they have the twofold attribute of the natural and the human sciences. The model "qi-yinyang-wuxing" originates on the one hand from the ancient practical observation of living phenomena, on the other hand it is has been restricted by the Chinese traditional way of thought. It describes relational reality not substantial reality. There is a famous proposition in Chinese medicine: "medicine is meaning (/concept/ opinion)", it illustrates that Chinese medical theory and practice has the speciality of subjective thought, this is because of an objectivity that is higher than objectivity, it is a raising of objectivity as a whole, and it has a strong humanist thought tendency/ sentiment. In those times it was impossible for man to find out about the biological "substantial structure" that was verified some thousand years later. Therefore, the concepts of Chinese medical studies could not be established starting from the level of cells, molecules and genes, but just like nowadays Chinese medical basic research needs to start from there, and bring the biological fundament to light. During the last few decades, the studies had the goal to find the "substantial basis", demanded a turn to objectivity, standardization, to measurement, and used the means of concrete evidence and experiment. Even though they have achieved many results, it has to be accepted that many results contradict each other, some take a part for the whole, and generalize from isolated incidents: others list one but omit thousands, so they are far from being complete. In my opinion, the basic reason of this situation is that they are not clear about the concepts of Chinese medical studies and the essence of their model.

Fritz Wallner

Comment to Zhang Qicheng's Contribution

Zhang's contribution is wonderful and rich. There are a number of aspects which are very close to my own scientific insights. Especially at the end of the contribution there are important advices in order to consider the difference of Western research and Chinese medicine. I would like to emphasize on the topic of intercultural research and discuss some insights from the field of philosophy of science as well as some advices for this research.

1. Summary and Comment: the peculiarities of TCM

The first aspect I want to focus is Zhang's reference to the basic problem of translation. It is nonsense for Chinese medicine to translate the original texts in the usual way word by word or even sentence by sentence. Instead you have to translate the cultural connotations. In this respect all translations into English and German are deficient. If we look for instance to the concept of "Qi", we will see that it is physical and functional, temporally extensional, metaphysical and explanatory. No Western thinker, not even Hegel, could form all this into just one idea. Let us summarise this idea of Qi again with this formula that functions – because we have to find a way for the translation of cultural connotations. We should keep in mind in respect to Qi that one cultural connotation must not be separated.

There is a side-aspect of Zhang's lecture I like very much: the reference to religion. My own research on cultural differences, on frameworks of culture and their structure showed the importance of the structural influence of religion. E.g., in the Christian religion morality and religion are separated – hence everyone can be moral without being religious. In Confucianism it is not separated, both go together.

Zhang's demonstration of the Yin-Yang as a demonstration of the visualisation of thinking was very impressive. According to my own research this thought of 'visualisation of thinking', 'thinking by observing' is central for understanding the procedure of Chinese medicine. I have to make a philosophical summary in one ore two sentences in this respect. We could say Yin-Yang is the principle of opposite while it is mutually opposed and mutually harmonious: Harmony by opposition, opposition by harmony – there is no harmony without opposition. This is an expressive example for my thesis concerning the Chinese culture reading that Chinese culture is an 'including culture' (in difference to the Western 'exculuding culture').

Zhang's scientific results on Wuxing (five basis, five elements, and five types of one principle) are very important. Wuxing and Qi together can be understood as the reality of relation and function. Functions are as real as substances. This is an important aspect for another type of research that is now coming up in Europe: the research on traditional European medicine, the so called TEM (Traditional European Medicine). In TEM exists the idea of the elements, too. There are also theories about five elements in this TEM. It is often stated that these five elements in TEM differ from the Chinese five elements, what I consider as nonsense. The important aspect is that the former European doctors, too, were good observers, but they lacked the Chinese framework. Therefore their theory is different from the Chinese Wuxing-thinking. According to my scientific work it is to mention that insights into methodology have to be emphasized. And these methodological insights can stimulate the research on TEM.

I have to confess that I admire the linguistics and ontology of the model Qi, Yin-Yang and Wuxing. It offers relational reality and not substantial reality. As cultures are not closed systems, there are several attempts in Europe to direct the thinking to the 'relational reality'. But these attempts are done by outsiders and are forgotten by the majority because they simply don't fit to our culture. E.g., Alfred Whitehead and his well known colleague Bertrand Russell wrote *Principia Mathematica*. As a side aspect of this important book about the logics of mathematics Whitehead developed a „theory about the reality as events". I mention this because this might be interesting for the communication in the future. But he was an outsider in Europe. I would like that we don't forget this interesting connection – a mathematician like Whitehead invented a theory of the events stepping out from the theory of substances.

Zhang's comments on the fundamental difference between Chinese and Western medicine in research and in practise are very important. The argument that the Western medicine always must kill is radical, but I like it very much.

2. Essential differences of Occidental and traditional Chinese medicine

As a second step I want to characterise the differences and peculiarities of the scientific and medical systems of Western medicine and traditional medicine as well as their typical ways of healing. Both medical systems – the European and the Chinese – treat people successfully. In general these both medical systems share the goal (health), but this similarity gets lost if you consider the details. Western medicine is defined as a natural science like physics, chemistry and biology since about 200 years. Chinese medicine is not a natural science in this sense. Chinese medicine is directed to nature, but it doesn't fulfill the Western definition of being a natural science.

Western medicine works like Western science refering to nature by lifting out specific qualities and making up theories about the facts gained by that abstraction. By this procedure Western medicine gets the concept of disease defined as specific quality that is not good for the body. In difference to this type of scientific work Chinese medicine observes the relation between nature and human being. Chinese medicine does not abstract, it does not lift out qualities of nature – instead of the Western procedure Chinese medicine connects qualities. Western science can be understood as a way of theory application to a specific situation of the human body – applying theory. The Chinese way is to interpret relations that do not work. In Europe this Chinese way is called "hermeneutics", the art of interpretation. Chinese medicine interprets a situation of the body and enforces the possibilities of the body for self-healing by this way. Chinese medicine can be described as healing by understanding. Western medicine instead is healing by fighting against diseases. In Chinese medicine there is no fight – there is the aim of understanding the way in that the wheels of the body go (so to speak). Chinese medicine is closer to the Western so called "geisteswissenschaften" or humanities. Clearly Chinese medicine is not a "geisteswissenschaft".

Zhang stresses the definition of Chinese medicine as meaning. The Austrian philosopher Ludwig Wittgenstein comes very close to this when he says: The world consists of propositions. You must understand that this phrase is literally nonsense. Clearly this is not a proposition, but it means that the linguistic structure is subjective and objective together; or we only can understand objects if we understand linguistic structure while we cannot understand linguistic structures if we don't have objects. In Western medicine subjective reasoning is without importance, in Chinese medicine subjectivity has another sense. The Western scientist makes observations, and by abstracting from his subjective experience he gains so called objective data. The Western scientist resembles an observing machine. This idea is strange for TCM. The observation in TCM is always done in specific ways, in subjective ways done by the master. According to TCM experience is to follow the master's way.

3. Research on cultural differences: building bridges

3.1 The theoretical approach of a cooperation: a neutral standpoint

How is it possible for Chinese medicine to cooperate with Western medicine? Since it is not possible to cooperate by adopting the methodology of Western medicine (this way is equal to the destruction of TCM) or by adopting the TCM methodology (an idea that is not proposed that often), we must find a standpoint outside of Western and Chinese medicine.

I recently had a discussion with an open-minded Western doctor. He considered Yin-Yang as an idea that is wonderful and good, but Wuxing, five bases (five elements) as a speculation. If Westerners are free to take out what they understand of TCM and neglect what they don't understand, then the Chinese cultural heritage is lost in the next 20 or 30 years.

At this point we also can answer the question: Why do scientists from Chinese medicine and Chinese pharmacology cooperate with scientists from the field of philosophy and philosophy of science? Why should philosophers assist the intercultural research of the two named medical systems? Because philosophy and philosophy of science offers the named platform by which you can observe both medical systems from a neutral standpoint, in a neutral way, neither involved in one, nor involved in the other one.

But what is this platform like and what concept and ideas does it offer? The methodological concept I offer for this research is the approach of "Constructive Realism". It offers the concepts that can make the fundaments and implicit basic theoretical background of a research explicit and characterise its structure and peculiarity. Research is only possible under specific presuppositions. Therefore the results of a research program can only be true in respect to these presuppositions. We can assume that scientific truth is not independent from the framework of our thinking.

The position of Constructive Realism offers an ontology which can serve both cultures – Chinese culture and Western culture because the concept of microworlds offers a system of relations. What are "microworlds"? Let us shortly refer to the thoughts of the Vienna circle. The Vienna circle produced essential ideas in the field of philosophy of science until the discussion became absurd. According to my opinion the result of this long discussion of 30 or 40 years has one striking result. This striking result is that science constructs micro-worlds. The Vienna circle could not solve the problem of the empirical basis. It was a great idea but this idea does not work in respect to science. The Vienna circle also could not solve the problem of demarcation, of the border between science and not science. As we cannot find a clear concept of the empirical basis of science we must replace the idea of describing the world by science by the idea of constructing world models which are representing the world. This world model we name "micro-world".

I want to give you examples for a micro-world: one famous, important and interesting micro-world is the classical physics, classical mechanics or the mechanics of Sir Isaac Newton in physics in Western science. For comparison we must introduce some ideas of the Western science. Otherwise it does not make sense. A good example is Newtonian mechanics. We could name it also the system of moving things. A micro-world is the Newtonian system of moving things. I also want to give you an example for a TCM-micro-world: one TCM-micro-world is the system of meridians.

Micro-worlds are real systems of relations. They avoid the temptation of mechanical management of the world which is typical for Western thinking. The temptation of mechanical management is to look at the body like a machine which can be repaired. Therefore in the Western world there is a serious obstacle against an integrative medicine. Therefore there is the tendency to make this division between the mechanics of the world which is scientific and the esoteric, unscientific thinking of the world. It's a strange thing that in the Western world people take Chinese medicine to the field of esoteric very often – but this can be understood as nonsense.

Constructive Realism states that science can be understood as artificial and constructed systems of data and propositions; that science is to consider as a constructed "micro-world", a world that selects and reduces qualities in certain respects and that is important for our thinking and our actions as well.

In that sense we can differ between two essential und fundamental dimensions of scientific work: "realität" and "wirklichkeit". Those notions are German words. I seriously insist to use the German words and not to translate them because both would mean "reality" in English what blurs an essential differentiation. "Realität" describes the scientific micro-worlds, the world that is constructed by the selection and exclusion of qualities of the object, a process that is guided by theory. On the other hand "wirklichkeit" describes the genuine world, the world that depicts the fundament for realität and the basis for the selection and reduction. This is the world that we are living with and that keeps us alive (for example when it feeds us).

Now let us focus on the relation of those worlds and ask the question whether and in what way they are connected: As it was already mentioned those "micro-worlds" or "realitäten" in general are to consider as artificial worlds, as results of scientific actions. Concerning the relation of realität to wirklichkeit we have to propose that in any case there is a reference of realität to wirklichkeit as far as the constructions are selecting and excluding the qualities of wirklichkeit. Thus we have to name two characteristics of this relation: first the reference and second the reduction of the manifoldness of wirklichkeit. This also means that we have to reject the idea that the scientific systems and their data systems were identical to wirklichkeit respectively that wirklichkeit was structured in the same way as the scientific systems.

Let us apply these arguments on the relation of Western and Chinese science: Based on the insights of Constructive Realism we can consider science the way that it is not in correspondence with nature while science is a job constructing models which are somehow in a specific way connected with nature. The main point of the results in the last 50 years of research on the structure of Western science is that science is a manifold-ness of constructions of our reference to the world. We have many different constructions of these references. Some of them are compatible, some of them are incompatible. Therefore there is one thing you should consider: There is manifoldness of perceiving the world, not just one way and not just one solution – as the Western science usually believes.

In the last 15 years we have seen another aspect which was so hard to understand for European scientists especially for European philosophers of science: that science also is dependent from culture. That means that science is guided by cultural convictions. Therefore it is fair to contend that we have a Western science or European science. This is a term we use in difference to a Chinese science, in difference to sciences or scientific attempts of other cultures. It is fair because in this case we contend that there is not only one way to make a structure of the world and that there are different ways to form those structures of the world in an intellectual manner.

Based on this understanding of science and the named ontological concept – the thoughts of "micro-worlds", of "realität", "wirklichkeit", their relation to each other and the thought of the different possibilities of constructing micro-worlds – we have the theoretical basis to consider both medical systems as independent and incompatible; as well as we have the theoretical fundament to observe both medical systems from a neutral standpoint, in a neutral way, neither involved in one, nor involved in the other one.

At the end I would like to stress one thing that I focused in my last speech at the Academy of Medical Sciences. It is a little bit difficult to understand but I think it is going with your ideas that we must put together the field of ruling and the field of understanding. What you have expressed about Yin-Yang was a wonderful construct in the field of understanding but not in the field of ruling. There is no ruling in the Western sense. Therefore my formula is to make the understanding ruling and the rules understood.

3.2 The way of a cooperation and methodological mistakes

I strictly recommend avoiding simple comparisons between Western medicine and TCM. If you find similarities and try to understand one of the two medical systems, you take the wrong way. My recommendation is to stress the differences. Take the idea or some ideas of one system into the context of the other system to make understandable how different these ideas are. To give you one example: false diagnosis in TCM and false diagnosis in Western medicine. Do not compare them! There are some similarities. Take the false diagnosis in TCM into the system of Western medicine and you will see that it will destroy the system of Western medicine. By this way you will understand the difference of these two systems. By this way you can learn the importance of qualitative reasoning in difference to quantitative reasoning.

Another mistake which is very common is the reference to common ideas or the attempt to go to a universalized, to a common medical reasoning between TCM and Western medicine; the reference to common ideas, to ideas which are at the first glance common in both systems.

Gertrude Kubiena

Teaching Traditional Chinese Medicine outside China – A Challenge for Teachers

Western TCM-teachers for Western students have to fight a multi-front-battle: There are several linguistic problems: ambiguous or even wrong interpretations of Chinese terms, many synonyms, which are indiscriminately used by different authors and books. Further there are two sorts of preoccupation by Western students: One part thinks TCM is a sort of esoteric phantasm and it is not necessary to study hard and exactly: The second preoccupation claims on the cultural difference, which makes it almost impossible to concentrate on the subject for this – fortunately small – group. To be able to digest the stuff and even to apply it practically seems impossible to them. This and the limited capacity of the human brain make it necessary to use the technique of strangification to make TCM "light and easy" and encourage Western students. It is not hopeless, it is learnable! And it is worth learning because a combined knowledge of modern Western and Traditional Chinese Medicine enriches not only one's therapeutic horizon but as well one's personality-development. It is like getting an additional eye for viewing the Chinese world of health and disease besides the Western one.

1. Introduction

Concerning so called complementary medical methods Austria is relatively open-minded. 15th Sept 2004 the Austrian Board of MDs even decided to establish a diploma "Complementary Medicine – Chinese Diagnostics and Herbal Therapy". In contrast to the United States, UK, Germany or France, in Austria practicing medicine is restricted to medical doctors. So the students of TCM are MDs, medical students, a few veterinaries and some pharmacists.

That means that our TCM-students either still are or have been indoctrinated for at least five to six years with the theories of Western medicine as the only true and valid. A great part of the students' brain – first of all the memory system – is fatigued by the study of human/veterinary medicine or pharmacology. The rest of the brain has to be activated later, when practice of medicine starts. The university gives wonderful security: There is a – not to be called in question – scientific basis, there is a state of the art. That there may be a different approach towards physiology and pathology is strictly denied. Nevertheless – all of us know that everything may change from one second to the other if there is a new finding, e.g. the discovery of the blood-circulation system, microorganisms, X-rays, antibiotics etc. Nevertheless we learn that medicine is science. So, for the Western MD, philosophers like Fritz Wallner, are shocking as they doubt the scientificy of medicine. Anyway, teaching TCM for Western students is a challenge for Western TCM-teachers.

In more than 20 years of teaching TCM I learned that there are three main problems:

- the cultural difference between modern Western and Traditional Chinese Medicine,
- ambiguous translations and even misinterpretations of TCM-terms and synonyms,
- the limitation of the capacity of memory.

2. Discussion

2.1 The cultural difference between modern Western and Traditional Chinese Medicine

Any of the two medical systems is based on its contemporary theory of science. The background of TCM for some people – especially very conventional modern MDs – gives rise to complete rejection, for others – and their amount grows continually – it is totally fascinating.

One day the chairman of Austria's highest medical board – a very conventional Western MD and old friend of mine – asked me if one could not simply skip the background of TCM. Unfortunately I took the physiology of the "Chinese spleen" as an example to explain why it is important to know the TCM-physiology otherwise it would not be logical why we needle acupoints of the spleen and stomach channel to influence the metabolic system. His reaction: "Nonsense! Nowadays we know everything about the functions of the spleen!" There was not a trace of readiness to notice the key point – the different approach to physiology and pathology of two medical systems. TCM was measured with the measure of modern Western Medicine. This is as absurd as to measure length with gram.

Some of our students close their mind and react like my old friend; but the majority is open minded and fascinated by TCM. Many of them – especially nowadays students – never learned to use their sense-organs. The older MDs are frustrated by bureaucracy, endless lists of laboratory findings and lack of time for individual treatment. Although TCM is an absolute concise and logical system it is as well a sensual medicine! It does not only allow, no, it requires the observance of feelings!

And so the first challenge for Western TCM-teachers is to make clear to the students that TCM-background is not an esoteric phantasm but a bony hard system, which is logical in itself and based on findings with the sense-organs. Summarising findings – the signs and symptoms – results in defining a certain pattern or syndrome. For each pattern TCM has very clearly defined therapeutic principles, which are to be followed. In this respect TCM always has been as strict as modern Western Medicine with its state of the art.

2.2 Ambiguous translations and even misinterpretations of TCM-terms and synonyms

When I started to study Chinese Medicine – like almost everybody in the West with acupuncture – my teacher forbade us students to deal with the TCM-background. The reason was the lack of qualified translations of the classical literature. My teacher studied acupuncture in France and with French books. As TCM came to France via Vietnam one can imagine how the translations were like: simply ununderstandable. Although things have changed since then there are still a lot of ambiguous interpretations, I dare say even misinterpretations, which make the understanding of TCM more difficult than necessary.

Some very simple examples:
Yuan qi – yuán qì 原气 is translated source qi or congenital qi or primary qi or essential qi in the kidney.

Xue – xué 穴 is translated "point", but it does not mean "point". Xué 穴 means "cave, hole, lair" and "acupuncture point". The pictogram shows what an acupuncture point is like: a door, covered by a lid – a closed entrance, which can be opened by needling.

Jing-luo – jïng luò 经 络 is frequently translated "meridian". The term creates the imagination of a fictive two-dimension line system, but means a three-dimensional channel-network.

Wu shu xue – wû shø xué 五输 穴 five transport points: "Antike Punkte" (antique points) is the German term. This says absolutely nothing about their function namely the transportation of vital energy qi.

He xue – hé xué 合穴, the transport point close to elbow / knee is translated "he-sea-point" but hé 合 does not mean "sea", but "to close, unite".

In German the mother and child points are named "Tonisierungs- und Sedativpunkte" (reinforcing and reducing points), neglecting their interrelation according to the five elements – in contrast to the English expression.

Qi jing ba mai – qí jïng bã mài 七 经 八 脉 is frequently translated "extra meridians". This implies that the respective channels are out of order, in Chinese the expression is related to the most original channel-like structures with extraordinary potency.

Xi ze qu huan – xî zé qì huãn is a classical statement concerning joy – xi xî 喜, one of the seven emotions, which is necessary for normal movement of qi but may become pathogenic if there are Severe, continuous or abruptly occurring emotional stimuli. The above mentioned quotation is translated in a very different way:

- The Classified Dictionary of Traditional Chinese Medicine quotes: 'Excessive joy makes the qi sluggish'.
- Liu Yanchi: joy (heart) → if normal: 'encourages circulation of qi and blood. Over-joy → scattering of heart qi, inability to concentrate'.
- Chinese Acupuncture and Moxibustion: 'joy causes the qi to move slowly.

These are very contradictory translations or rather interpretations. As well different authors attach different emotions with different interior organs, see the list on page 79. This makes teaching TCM very difficult for Western teachers.

2.3 The limitation of the capacity of memory

As the brains of Western TCM-students have already a sort of overload from the university and from the attempt to practice evidence based medicine – even the open minded find it difficult to keep all these strange things, imported from a foreign world, in mind. Anyway: Six years of indoctrination with Western Medicine are hemming on the way as well as preoccupation in two directions: Some students claim on the idea that TCM is only a sensual medicine and therefore it is not necessary to study for TCM as hard as for Western Medicine. Another part cannot come clear with the medical concept of a foreign world and builds up a sort of brain-blocking resistance.

There starts the next challenge for Western teachers for Western students: Resistance must be broken or at least softened. And it is absolutely important to bring the students to serious studying. To help them to understand things and to keep them in mind the TCM-teacher must give associations with familiar ideas to his students.

To understand TCM-pathomechanisms and TCM-pathology we first need a definition of health in TCM. Health means:

- balance between yin and yang
- sufficient amount of vital substances
- harmony between the five phases
- harmony between microcosm (human being) and macrocosm
- free flow of qi and blood

Disease is – of course – a sort of deviation of health caused by various reasons. The Etiology of Diseases (pathogenesis) reads:

- Six exogenous pathogenic factors corresponding not only with the bioclimatic factors but as well with microorganisms
- Seven emotions, considered the main reason of interior diseases: Western students are fascinated by the idea that TCM already thousands of years ago recognized the importance of psychical and mental influences on physical health. In the West this idea spread but in the 20th century!
- improper diet: a major problem in the West; we recently exported it to China with McDonalds
- over strain, too much work
- lack of physical exercise: "internetitis"

- traumatic injuries
- bites by insects or wild animals
- stagnated blood and phlegm fluid: very difficult to understand for Western students!

We suppose that for Chinese students many of these ideas are familiar from childhood on. But first of all that's not true and second consider: For Western students *everything* is new and strange. And like we change a preponderance of yang in yin by tilting it over we strangify the strange to make it digestible for Western brains.

3. TCM-Basics

3.1 Yin and Yang

To explain yin and yang we can refer to a European tradition starting with Aristotle's (matter and form) and elaborated by Einstein: Material stuff and energy are identical. Anything has a yin- and a yang-aspect. E.g. we can see a car as a heap of sheet metal or as a moving vehicle. If the stuff (yin) is o.k. the function (yang) will as well be o.k. If you overload your car with tins, tents, mother in law etc., it will be difficult to climb up a mountain road because to much yin impedes yang. If you don't replenish fuel (yin) your car will not move (yang). If you always drive full speed (yang) and don't replenish cooling fluid and oil (yin) your car will get too hot (yang) and several parts will be damaged as yang consumes yin.

When your car is already old the stuff is corroded and it will start to leak out water or oil – a good example to give an idea what jing deficiency is like. Back to yin and yang: The implication of transformation can be clarified by the relation of food and energy or even the production of a car: That yïn 阴 and yáng 阳 as well stand for transformation and contrast is well known. That nowadays feminists are not delighted with the following statement is out of discussion: Yang is the male principle of light and life, and Yin is the female principle of darkness and death (see Veith 1949, pp.97-253).

3.2 First steps in pattern differentiation: Eight Principles – ba gang – bā gāng 八 纲

For the differentiation of yin-yang-imbalances TCM uses the pattern differentiation according to the Eight Principles – ba gang – bā gāng 八 纲. What is mostly neglected is that – exploring an Eight-Principle-Pattern – the questions should be listed up in a certain order to come to a satisfying result:

The first question is always: Interior or Exterior? If there is an Exterior pattern the second question has to be for Cold or Heat? Why? Because an exterior pattern is defined as presence of a pathogen in the exterior. The presence of a pathogen means presence of something unnecessary, which does not belong into the body. And this is Excess/Repletion. Nevertheless the question for Repletion or Depletion has to be clarified finally because there may be underlying deficiency of one of the vital substances. The usual expressions are a little bit upsetting: Exterior Excess/Repletion versus Exterior Deficiency/Depletion pattern. Anyway, the differentiation has to be done as the therapeutic approach differs according to the actual pattern.

For an Interior pattern the second question has to be about Excess or Deficiency and only the third question asks for Cold or Heat, as any interior pattern develops one of the both conditions in the course of time.

It is incredible how difficult it is to train students to recognise and memorize the simplest symptoms: So simple it seems to answer the question: "Talking about eight principles: What does the color red indicate?" The correct answer is: "Heat" – what else? But 50 per cent of the beginners will answer – even after several trainings: "Excess".

3.3 The vital substances

To explain the relation between jīng 精, qì 气 and shén 神 I use the money in the bank for essence – jīng 精: It is good to have it there but as long as it is in the bank – where is the fun? To transform money into joy it must be activated (e.g. by using the cash machine) to transform it into qi. Whereas jīng 精 is a concentrated, indolent substance, qì 气 is like champagne – sparkling, vitalizing, moving, warming – a juice for life! Finally from champagne arises a gas, comparable with shén 神. As a sort of gas, shén 神 is very light and easy movable, e.g. by acupuncture. Therefore one has to be careful if treating psychoses as outdoor patients.

3.4 Jing, qi, spleen and stomach

It lasts a while until students understand the concept of qi and the important role of stomach and spleen within the qi-production: To stay alive we have to breath, drink and eat. Whatever we eat or drink – it will be transformed by the spleen into our personal flesh, blood, energy. This is so because all of us are borne with a sort of ground-plan, anchored in a substance we got from our parents – the congenital essence – jing – jīng 精. During the course of life this congenital jing is used up because it is gradually transformed into the primary or source qi – yuán qì 原气. The yuán qì 原气 adapts any transformative action of any input from the exterior to the body belonging to. One may compare this congenital jīng 精 respectively the yuán qì 气 to the DNA and its functions.

The "input" – food and beverages – is primarily processed by the stomach, which chops and crashes it and so adapts the gǔ qì 谷气. The latter is then transformed by the spleen, which can be compared with a refinery, to become clear qi – qīng qì 清气. Qing qi is still rather substantial. If we look to the old character for qì 氣 we can very well note, that there are two components: damp – air, and rice – food.

From this qīng qì 清气 one part is sent up directly to the lung to produce the actual warmth and defense, another part is sent to the heart to color it red and so produce blood. A third part is offered to the ancestors, who are sitting behind the sternum and may be taken as another expression for immune system. TCM talks about zong qi – zōng qì 宗气. If the stuff is accepted it will become the true qi – zhen qi – zhēn qì 真气, with two aspects: protective qi – wei qi – wèi qì 卫气 against pathogenic qi – xie qi – xié qì 邪气 from the ambiente; the perfectly clean part finally becomes ying qi – yíng qì 营气. Ying qi, which circulates in the channels, is called jīng luò zhī qì 经络之气; talking about the ying qi which is nourishing the interior organs it is called zàng fǔ zhī qì 脏腑之气.

These different aspects of the yíng qì 营气 frequently upset our students. The clarifying sentence: Coca Cola can be sold in bottles or in tins, but it is Coca Cola.

Another important aspect is that defense is not only performed by the wei qi. If that were like this we would have no chance against evils if the wei qi failed to defeat them. There is defense on different levels and all of these defensive energies are summarised under the expression upright qi –zhèng qí 正气, which implies:

- the most superficial level – wèi qì 卫气
- the level of the zang fu – zāng fǔ zhǐ qì 脏 腑 之气
- the most profound level – yuán qì 原气

3.5 Harmony and disharmony expressed by the Five Elements – wǔ xíng 五行

The mother-child-relation of the five elements is so obvious that it is astonishing why students sometimes have difficulties to keep it in mind. Maybe that comes from the usual translation of "xing" by "elements". "Phases" is by far the better expression because the expression "elements" gives an association with the four elements of the Greek philosophy. On the other hand "phases" implies the transformation of one into the other and clarifies the consumption of the mother by the child.

To explain xiāng kè 相 克 and xiāng wǔ 相 侮 I try to give examples of everyday's life: First of all the students are instructed to picture the five phases in order of a circle and to start with the most logical relation, namely water controlling fire. They get a picture of a fire brigade struggling against a fierce fire to clarify the relation between control – xing ke and resistence – xiang wu.

Fire controlling metal: Metal can only be worked by heating it with fire. This is another good example for the relation between control and resistance respectively over control and rebellion: lead can easily be melted by a candle's flame, stainless steel is much more resistant – rebellious and requires strong fire. Too strong fire will even burn metal – this corresponds to over control.

Metal controlling wood is demonstrated by a saw, whereby everybody can understand the different resistance of pine wood and iron wood. That wood has to control earth – keep it in its place – everybody can understand if looking to a picture of severe earth erosion. And this picture leads very quickly to the last control-rebellion-relation: Earth has to control water, once more to keep it in its place. The strongest earth cannot control a flood disaster.

Regarding the translation of the expression ke – kè 克 some doubts arise: Is, what we interpret, actually the meaning of kè? Once we interpret it as limitation, another time as subduing and still another time as making soft and treatable. The Concise English-Chinise Chinese-English Dictionary offers the following translations:

1. restrain
2. overcome, subdue, capture
3. set a time limit
4. gram

To know the relations between the five phases is only a first step on the thorny way of a Western TCM-student: Now follows the problem to keep in mind all the related ideas associated with each of the five phases and to integrate them into every day's practice. E.g. when we know that the fire controls metal, we can transfer this relation to heart controlling lung. This is logical, also for Western brains, because insufficiency of the heart causes lung edema. Less logical is the relation between metal and fire if we transfer it to the human body: This means that the lung has to control the liver. The only explanation to agree with is for me the relation between the soul of the lung – the soft and very sensitive corporeal soul of the lung – pò 魄 and the combative and somewhat animal-like soul of the liver – hun – hún 魂. The liver is associated with emotions in general and anger especially. An explosive temper may cause difficulties to some personalities of the higher management. So they start to study breathing techniques to subdue their rising yang. Some of them become so soft in the course of time that they only speak in quotations any more.

Is that now only strangification or has it a real background from the TCM-point of view?

3.6 Stagnation, its various reasons, and therapeutic approaches

It is easy to understand that a traumatic injury or tough substances (among which the exterior pathogens are as well summarised) in the channels can cause stagnation. Not so easy is it to understand why deficiency of a vital substance as well can cause stagnation. For clarifying I use a very ordinary picture, namely a WC. Obstruction can be caused by tough substances as well as by lack of qì 气 – not enough pressure on the rinsing button; lack of blood – xué 血 or yīn 阴暗 – not enough water in the rinsing box; or lack of yáng 阳– freezing in winter; or by deficiency of jīng 精– leaching out of the rinsing water.

Understanding the various pathomechanisms of stagnation makes obvious that very different therapeutic approaches are required. The mere presence of an impediment requires its removal. This is the domain of acupuncture! But only as long as the obstructing substance is soft enough to be moved by qì 气. That means that acupuncture will give no satisfactory effect there is a tough substance like flame or static blood. Even aggravation is predictable because acupuncture moves qi and if there is a sort of stone in the way pain will become worse. So – what can we do? Before we use acupuncture we have to dissolve the hard masses with chemistry – herbal therapy. The same idea is valid for the lack of substances like blood or yin: Acupuncture does not produce substances immediately; it only can stimulate the producers of the substances – spleen, stomach and kidney.

Nevertheless it is astonishing that mere acupuncture can improve yin-deficiency-symptoms, e.g. in menopausal syndrome. This happens because with acupuncture we reduce yang and so stop it consuming yin. That means we bring both – yin and yang – to a level, which is usually lower than the normally required. Herbal therapy gives by far better and steadier results.

3.7 Acupuncture according to time –五 运 六 气 针 灸 疗 法 – wǔ-yún-liù-qì-zhēn-jiǔ-liáo-fǎ

This is a very special approach but effective acupuncture method. There are several methods to needle according to the time.

One of the various theories says that the time applicable for 灵 龟 八 法 – líng-guǐ-bā-fǎ can only be calculated according to the stellar time. That means that the genuine time unit of an hour is not 60 minutes but a little bit more, namely one minute and 45 seconds. Does the system of Chinese of the available turning tables refer to this recognition? May be we should discuss this very specific subject in a following special symposium.

List of abbreviations of the table (see next side):
Class: Classified Dictionary of Traditional Chinese Medicine
CAM: Chinese Acupuncture and Moxibustion
Liu Yanchi: The Essential Book of Traditional Chinese Medicine

Footnote of the table:
1   Feit/Zmiewski: Support = dejected, sorrowful countenance

汉字	pinyin	Wise-man	joy (heart)	Class.			CAM	Liu Yanchi	F/Z
喜	1 xǐ	joy (heart)	joy (heart)	喜则气缓	xǐ zé qi huǎn	Excessive joy makes the qi sluggish	joy causes the qi to move slowly	joy (heart) → normal: encourages qi and blood circulation. Over-joy → scattering of heart qi; inability to concentrate	joy (heart)
怒	2 nù	anger (liver)	anger, rage (liver)	怒则气上	nù zé qi shàng	rage causes the liver qi to flow adversely upward	anger causes the qi to rise up	anger (liver)	anger (liver)
悲	3 bēi	sorrow (lung)	sorrow (lung)	悲则气消(-)Qi	bēi zé qi xiāo	sorrow makes the qi (of the lung) consumed	grief drastically consumes qi	grief (lung) → dejection or stagnation of qi	support ↑ (lung)
忧	4 yōu	anxiety (lung)	melancholy (lung)	忧则气郁	nù zé qi yù	melancholy makes the qi stagnated	melancholy drastically consumes qi	sadness (lung) → lung qi stagnation	anxiety (lung or spleen)
思	5 sī	thought (spleen)	anxiety (spleen)	思则气结	sī zé qi jié	anxiety makes the qi depressed (often resulted in indigestion)	worry causes qi to stagnate	pensiveness (spleen) → depression and stagnation of qi	anxiety (lung or spleen)
恐	6 kǒng	fear (kidney)	fear (kidney)	恐则气下	kǒng zé qi xià	fear causes qi to sink (incontinence, seminal discharge)	fear causes qi to decline	fear (kidney) → kidney qi↓	fear (kidney)
惊	7 jīng	fright (kidney)	fright (kidney)	惊则气乱	jīng zé qi luàn	fright makes the qi (of the heart) disturbed	fright causes it to be deranged	fright (kidney) → heart qi "wander about, adhering to nothing"	fright (kidney)

Reference

Cheng Xinnong 1987, *Chinese Acupuncture and Moxibustion*, Beijing: Foreign Language Press.

Feit R. / Zmiewski P. 1989, *Acumoxa Therapy Volume I and II*, Brookline, Massachusetts: Paradigm Publications.

Flaws B. 1994, *Statements of Fact in Traditional Chinese Medicine*. Boulder:Blue Poppy Press, Inc.

Kaptchuk, Ted 2004, *The Web Has No Weaver. Understanding Chinese Medicine*. Palgrave Macmillan Copyright 1983.

Kubiena G. / Ramakers F. 2002, Bestzeitakupunktur Chronopunktur. Akupunktur der Meister nach der energetischen Zeit. Mit CD: *Computerprogramm zur Feststellung des aktuellen Qi-Flusses*, Wien-München-Bern: Verlag Wilhelm Maudrich.

Liangsheng Wu N. / Qi Wu A 1997, *Huang Di Nei Jing(Yellow Emperor´s Canon Internal Medicine)*,Beijing: Chinese Science and Technology Press.

Liu Yanchi 1988, *The Essential Book of Traditional Chinese Medicine. Volume I and II.*, New York: Columbia University Press.

Maoshing Ni, PH.D 1995, The Essential Text of Chinese Health and Healing – The Yellow Emperor´s Classic of Medicine.,*A New Translation of the Neijing Suwen with Commentary*, Shambala, Boston and London.

Pekinger Fremdspracheninstitut, Abteilung für Deutsch 1985, *Neues Chinesisch - Deutsches Wörterbuch*, Beijing: Shangwu yin Verlag.

Van Nghi, Nguyen 1977,*Hoang Ti Nei King So Ouenn*,Uelzen:Medizinisch Literarische Verlagsgesellschaft mbH.

Veith Ilza 1972(old edition 1949), *The Yellow Emperor's Classic of Internal Medicine*, Universitiy of California Press.

Wang Hua and Chen Xingjian(eds) 1992, *Chinese-English Dictionary of Acupuncture and Moxibustion,* Hubei Science and Technology Press, Sanlian Bookstore of Hong Kong.

Wiseman N. 1995, *English-Chinese Chinese-English Dictionary of Chinese Medicine*, Changsha: Hunan Science and Technology Press.

Wiseman N. / Ellis A. 1985, *Fundamentals of Chinese Medicine*, Brookline, Massachusetts: Paradigm Publications.

Xie Zhu-Fan / Lou Zhi-Cen (eds)1994,*Classified Dictionary of Traditional Chinese Medicine*, Beijing: New World Press.

Xinhua Dictionary (1990), Beijing: The commercial Press.

Zhao Tangshou 1992, *New German-Chinese Dictionary*, Beijing: Peking University Press.

Zhao Tangshou, *Chinesisch - Deutsch, Deutsch – Chinesisch* (2 Bände), Peking University Press (Beijing), Verlag Ute Schiller (Berlin), Yan Yuan Culture Industry LTD (K.K.).

Lan Fengli

Who Translated Huang Di Nei Jing: Influence of Translator's Subjectivities on Its Translation

Huang Di Nei Jing, also known as Nei Jing, comprising Su Wen and Ling Shu, is the earliest systematic and complete Chinese medical classic extant in China. It is not only the breeding ground of the fundamental theories of TCM, but also an important component part of excellent cultural heritage of China. It has been guiding the development of TCM for over 2000 years. Up till present, it is still regarded as the prime classic of "the Four Great Classics" of TCM, and is a required course for TCM learners. As Donald Harper said, it is "the essential reference for ancient Chinese medicine and a valuable to research on early Chinese civilisation".

In the years between 1925 and 2007, eleven translated versions of Huang Di Nei Jing (including translation of Su Wen, or Ling Shu, or both) have been got published, which become a unique, splendid, valuable and rare case in the history of English translation of TCM ancient classics. There are great differences between these translations which have emerged in different historical periods.

How to evaluate the immense variety of translations? The highest appraisal for a translation can not go beyond that "the translation is true to the original, accords with the standard of 'faithfulness', 'clarity', and 'elegance'" or that "the translation vividly reproduces the meanings, connotations and charms of the original". And then, which translation deserves such appraisals? Is it fair to pioneers of Nei Jing translation? Of course, it is also very important to compare different translated versions of Nei Jing, to judge which one is good or which one is bad, i.e. "Prescriptive Translation Criticism Methodology". Here, I just want to say that research on translation only from the aspect of language and the yardstick of "faithfulness" will inevitably hide the translation subject from view, and will be unable to display translator's cultural creativity.

Then, who is the translation subject? There are about four answers to the question in the translation circle: (1) the translator is the translation subject; (2) the author and the translator are the translation subject; (3) the translator and the readers are the translation subject; (4) the author, the translator and the readers are the translation subject. Xu Jun said, "It's evident that we should consider the author's and readers' subjectivities when defining the translation subject, but in the center is the translator".[1]

Zha Mingjian, et al. tried to define "translator subjectivity" as follows: Translator subjectivity refers to the subjective initiative that the translator shows in translating in order to fulfill translation purpose, and is characterised by translator's awareness of culture, his or her moral character, as well as his or her cultural and aesthetical creativity.[2]

Nei Jing, the highest authority on TCM, is elegant and concise in language and comprehensive and profound in meaning. So, first of all, translation of Nei Jing should convey the knowledge and cultural connotations of TCM, just like translation of scientific and technological works. So, translator subjectivities of Nei Jing are not identical to that of literary works. Who translates?-translator subjectivities beyond reason (2001) by Douglas Robinson, an active and influential theoretician on translation in the Western world at the present time, aims at discussing various forces acting on translator, including translator's selfhood and interferences from outside world such as ideology and market-oriented economy.[3] Then, is the influence of "translator subjectivities" on translation equal to that of "various forces acting on translator" on translation? My answer is yes.

The thesis consists of four parts. The first part answers the question "who translated Huang Di Nei Jing" in the form of a table. The second part discusses the influence of translator subjectivities on translation of Nei Jing from such aspects as translator's academic background and structure of knowledge, translator's awareness of medical culture of the target language (English) and the intended readers. The third part probes into "the required accomplishments of the Nei Jing translator". The fourth part explores "who possess the required accomplishments of Nei Jing translation and how to translate it".

---

1   Xu Jun 2003, p.11
2   Zha Mingjian 2003, p.22
3   Lu Yuling 2004, p.56

1. Who Translated Huang Di Nei Jing?

The Huang Di Nei Jing Su Wen is the major part of Nei Jing for it is the foundation of TCM and contains a wealth of knowledge, including etiology, physiology, diagnosis, treatment and prevention of disease, as well as an in-depth investigation of such diverse subjects as ethics, psychology, astronomy, meteorology, chronobiology, and cosmology; while the Huang Di Nei Jing Ling Shu, also known as Classic of Acupuncture, discusses the distribution of meridians and acupuncture points, physiology and pathology of the zang fu organs, flow of wei-defense, qi, ying-nutrient, and blood, as well as application of needling techniques. And both contain 81 chapters, with two chapters of the Su Wen missing and subsequently added to it by later generation. The translated versions of the Su Wen are more than that of the Ling Shu.

Who translated Huang Di Nei Jing? Please see the table on pp.100f for details.

2. The Influence of Translator Subjectivities on Translation of Huang Di Nei Jing

As space is limited, it is impossible to discuss all the translators involved in the translation of Nei Jing. The thesis will only discuss several typical translators to clarify my views on the topic.

2.1 Translator's Academic Background and Structure of Knowledge

The concrete translating process is a vital link of the translation activity and the most outstanding aspect where translator subjectivities manifest. In the translating course of Nei Jing, translator has to develop three statuses, i.e. "reader", "interpreter", and "author" (the re-author that gives "the second life"to the original). As "reader", translator must read and understand Nei Jing; as "interpreter", translator must explain Nei Jing, exploring the ideas, contents, and aesthetic implications contained in it, and analyzing its historical, medical and cultural values, as well as its practical significance in the society; after the above-mentioned two steps, as "author", translator enters the stage of language transformation, paying attention to reproduce the ideas, contents, aesthetic implications, and linguistic style of Nei Jing with the target language. Whether translator can successfully develop the three statuses is mainly determined by translator's academic background and structure of knowledge.

TCM academic background and professional training in archaic Chinese, esp. medical archaic Chinese, are the basic requirements for correctly understanding Nei Jing. It is not easy whatsoever even for TCM students of China to understand Nei Jing, including undergraduates and graduates who have learned the course of Medical Archaic Chinese (yi gu wen, Archaic Chinese for TCM Purpose)!

Ilza Veith did not possess basic knowledge of TCM and archaic Chinese, so she always misinterpreted words through taking them too literally. Although English was her mother tongue and she was an expert historian of Western medicine, mistranslations caused by misunderstanding and misinterpreting Nei Jing could be found everywhere. For example:

Original Text: 帝曰：何以知其胜？岐伯曰：求其至也，皆归始春，未至而至，此谓太过，则薄所不胜，而乘所胜也，命曰气淫。(六节藏象论)

Veith's Translation: The Emperor asked: "How can one use this knowledge of their counteraction?"

Ch'I Po answered: "By seeking after the highest (good). Everything is restored at the beginning of spring. If people have not yet arrived at the highest (good) but nevertheless reach out for it, their action is called 'excessive'. Then there is carelessness everywhere, which can not be counteracted, and that which must be overcome is multiplied".[1]

Modern Interpretation: Huang Di asked, "How do we know when one will restrict another?" Qi Bo answered, "We will calculate the time of the arrival of the seasons from the first day of spring in the Chinese calendar. If the season has not arrived, but the corresponding weather is coming, which is known as excess. This excess will then violate the qi which normally restricts it (rebellion) and over-restrict the qi which is normally restricted by it (subjugation). This is called "qi yin", or reckless qi. (The translation accords with the modern interpretation by Guo Aichun.)

Except that "命曰气淫" was not translated, the whole paragraph of Veith's translation was mistranslated, esp. the underlined part was ex-

---

1 Veith 1972, p.137

tremely unreasonable. As we all know, "胜", "薄所不胜", and "乘其所胜" refer to "相克 (restrain or restrict)", "相侮 (reversely restrain or reversely restrict or rebel), and "相乘 (over-restrain or over-restrict or subjugate)" respectively.

It is worth to note that there was no modern interpretation of Nei Jing before the middle of the 20th century. So, the pioneers of Nei Jing translation like Ilza Veith had to understand and interpret Nei Jing written in archaic Chinese all by themselves. Following the establishment of TCM colleges throughout China since 1956, textual criticism, annotation, modern Chinese interpretation, and monographic studies on Nei Jing have been in full swing. Achievements have been got published one after another. So afterwards, translators can apply various research achievements on Nei Jing to the translating process. Actually, this is how facts stand. These achievements help translators solve many problems of understanding and interpreting Nei Jing. Therefore, as "reader" and "interpreter", almost all the translators of Nei Jing after Ilza Veith can correctly grasp the gist of the book.

But here other questions appear. For example, Wu Liansheng (father) and Wu Qi (son) are practitioners of TCM in America, but they do not have academic background of translation. So they translated the title of the book Huang Di Nei Jing into Yellow Empero's Canon Internal Medicine where "Empero" was misspelled and "of" should have been in between "Canon" and "Internal" but not. Actually, Huang Di 黄帝 is not an Emperor, Nei Jing does not refer to a Canon of Internal Medicine. According to the universally accepted explanation of the title Huang Di Nei Jing, it is suggested to be translated into Huang Di's Inner Classic.1 Wu Liansheng and Wu Qi translated the titles of chapters "刺热"、"刺疟"、"刺腰痛" of Nei Jing which share the same style and pattern into "Acupuncture for Treating the Febrile Diseases of the Viscera", "On Treating Malaria with Acupuncture", and "The Pricking Therapy for Lumbago of Various Channels" respectively, whose wordings, patterns, and styles are different from each other.2

Actually, TCM academic background and ability of understanding archaic Chinese are the lowest requirements for reading and interpreting Nei Jing. Besides, translator should possess some knowledge about bibliology,

---

1   Lan Fengli 2004, pp.175-77
2   Lan Fengli 2004, p.268

exegetics, textual criticism of TCM ancient texts so as to select a good edition as the original and understand annotations and commentaries of Nei Jing made through the ages... and so and so forth. And then, who possess such academic background?

Paul U. Unschuld (with degrees in Chinese studies, pharmacology, public health, and political sciences) has devoted himself to the study of history and science of TCM for over 30 years, and has distinguished himself as one of the world's leading authorities on the history of Chinese medicine. His books previously published include Medicine in China: A History of Pharmaceutics (1986), Nan-Ching – The Classic of Difficult Issues (1986), Medicine in China: A History of Ideas (1988), and Essential Subtleties on the Silver Sea (with Jurgen Kovacs, 1998), Medicine in China: Historical Artifacts and Images (2000), Forgotten Traditions of Ancient Chinese Medicine[1], etc.

The research project "English translation of Huang Di Nei Jing Su Wen" directed by Unschuld, initiated in 1988, has been going on until now through nearly 20 years of international cooperation at Institute for the History of Medicine of Munich University. In the prefatory remarks of the first publication of the project: Nature, Knowledge, Imagery in An Ancient Chinese Medical Text, the introductory book, Unschuld said, "The scope of the project was broad. It aimed at preparing the first complete, philologically sound English translation of the Su Wen together with a research apparatus that will be of help for future work on this text.

"I prepared a preliminary version of the translation to serve as a starting point for an extensive collaboration with Hermann Tessenow. His philological expertise contributed decisively to the result achieved, which will be published separately in three volumes. In addition, Tessenow has conducted a detailed analysis of the approximately three hundred fifty separate segments constituting the historical and structural layers of the Su Wen. The outcome of this study also will be published in several volumes".[2]

He also mentioned, "Zheng Jinsheng of the Research Institute of Medical History and Medical Literature of the China Academy of Traditional Chinese Medicine has stayed with us in Munich several times for ex-

---

1   It's a translation of Yi Xue Yuan Liu Lun by Xu Dachun in 1998.
2   Unschuld 2003, X

tended periods. He was of invaluable help in the compilation of the annotated bibliographies and of the survey of the doctrine of the five periods and six qi, published as an appendix to this volume."[1]

It is thus clear that Hermann Tessenow, a famous philologist in the West, and Zheng Jinsheng, a famous expert in medical history and medical literature of China, are the main collaborator of the Su Wen project. That is to say, Unschuld draws support from scholars of other related academic fields to make up shortcomings in his own structure of knowledge.

If translator is a lay person of the study of the Nei Jing, he or she may be completely unaware of the differences between different editions of the Nei Jing.

Before starting studying and translating Huang Di Nei Jing Su Wen, Unschuld carefully selected a famous good edition as the original, which was always ignored by other translators of the former times. As regards to the evolution of editions of the Su Wen, there are mainly 24-volume, 12-volume, 50-volume, 9-volume editions and newly annotated editions after the Ming Dynasty. Among them, the 24-volume editions refer to the editions inscribed according to the edition rearranged and annotated by Wang Bing, and Lin Yi, et al. (Jia You Original Text, 嘉祐原本), such as the edition inscribed by Gu Congde 顾从德. The Gu Congde edition, also known as the Ming edition (1550), was a famous good edition.[2] Unschuld selected a copy of Gu Congde edition, which is stored at the National Institute of TCM in Taibei, as the original.

Moreover, Unschuld took "the publication of annotated bibliographies of more than three thousand articles by Chinese authors of the twentieth century, as well as of more than six hundred monographs by Chinese and Japanese authors of past centuries" as the secondary sources for use. He said, "While our interpretation of the original is reflected in the English version, I have taken great care to quote as many consenting and dissenting Chinese and Japanese views as was feasible." [3] That is to say, Unschuld has combined study with translation closely by choosing and following what is good about the existing critical commentaries and various annotations made throughout the past ages on the text.

---

1   Unschuld 2003, XI
2   Ji Wenhui, Wang Damei 2000, pp.165-67
3   Unschuld 2003, X-XI

It is thus evident that translator's academic background and structure of knowledge exert greatest influence on the translating process and translating achievements (i.e. translation) of Nei Jing, are the most remarkable aspects in the translator subjectivities, and are the focus of discussion on translator subjectivities in the translation circle.

2.2. Translator's Awareness of Medical Culture of the Target Language (English) and the Intended Readers

Any translation is actuated by a certain cultural purpose. Anyway, translator always makes his or her decision on translation choice (which work he or she will translate), translation strategies (such as domestication or foreignization), and expected translation purpose according to his or her awareness of cultural needs of the target language. Translating process is a process of consultation between two cultures. In this sense, translator is the medium of two cultures. However, translator is not cultural neutral person whatsoever. Translator's cultural status and intention as well as influence of outside environment on translator will inevitably manifest in his or her translation choices, translation strategies, and the translation itself.

Awareness of readers is another aspect of translator's awareness of medical cultural needs of the target language. "Readers" are of vital significance in the "Receptive Aesthetics". Erwin Wolff put forward the concept of "intended reader", i.e. the readers whom the author designs his or her works for.[1] Wang Zuoliang, a former professor of Beijing Foreign Studies University, tirelessly exhorted translators at the end of a thesis Yan Fu's Intentions (严复的用心), "Attracting the intended readers in your mind is an important matter which should not be neglected by any translator".[2]

Although some short passages of the Nei Jing had been translated into Western languages and brief descriptions of its contents had appeared in various textbooks on Chinese medicine before 1949, no major part of it had ever before appeared in any Western language. So Ilza Veith was the first Western scholar who translated Nei Jing into Western language (English) and got her translation published. Ilza Veith was a medi-

1   Zhou Ning, Jin Yuanpu 1987, p.442
2   Wang Zuoliang 1989, p.42

cal historian. In the Preface, she said, "It should be realized, therefore, that the translation of this classic represents the approach of a medical historian rather than that of a Chinese philologist. It is hoped that this preliminary study will serve as a starting point for further work on the text, with more specific attention of its many linguistic problems."[1] That is to say, Veith laid special emphasis on the historical value of the Nei Jing.

Moreover, it was her intention to translate the entire Nei Jing, but after she translated the first 34 chapters of the Su Wen, she was convinced that "the first thirty-four chapters---the part here translated ---contain nearly all the basic ideas of the Nei Ching", what is actually meant that readers will get a full view of the entire Nei Jing if they read the translation of the chapters 1-34. Of course, all of the TCM workers will not agree with her. Veith also mentioned in the preface that her intended readers were the occidental medical historian.

It is thus clear that Ilza Veith introduced a general view of an ancient TCM classic of about 2000 years ago to the occidental medical historian from the approach of a medical historian, and hinted that she lacked professional knowledge on philology, i.e. she stressed bringing out "the actual contents of the work". But, anyway, she was willing to be a pioneer of the hard translating task.

In the 1940s, the modern Western medicine remained strong and self-sufficient in the West. English translation of TCM works, including English translation of TCM ancient classics, was in a very marginal position in the medical cultural system of the English speaking countries, which influenced or even determined Ilza Veith's cultural intention and selection, thus influencing her choice of translation strategies: stressing "acceptability" of the translation in the West. So she mainly adopted "domestication" translation strategy, using ready-made model of Western medicine indiscriminately, borrowing many Western medical terms to express unique TCM concepts. For example, she rendered "经，经脉" into "arteries (veins)", "经络系统" into "the vascular system", "天癸" into "menstruation", and so and so forth. Another example: translation of 脾 and 肾. Western medicine and TCM have extremely different viewpoints about the function of the spleen and kidneys. In Western medicine, the spleen is the

---

1 Veith 1972, XIV

largest endocrinal gland of the human body, whose main function is to get rid of the dead cells and fight infection; and the kidneys' main function is to maintain normal concentrations of the main constituents of blood, passing the waste matter into the urine. While in TCM, the main function of the Spleen is to transform and transport essence of the water and grain, i.e. a major organ for digestion, and the Kidneys govern growth, development and maturation of the male and female. When facing great differences between TCM and Western medicine, for the purpose of making the translation acceptable to the Western readers, i.e. the occidental medical historian, Ilza Veith knowingly and deliberately mistranslated 脾 and 肾 in Nei Jing: she rendered almost all of the "脾" in the original text into the "stomach", rendered the "肾" which involved governing male's growth, development, and maturation into "his testes (kidneys, 肾)".

In addition, for the purpose of making the readers truly enjoy reading and understanding Nei Jing and promoting interchange of medical cultures, Ilza Veith adopted many compensatory measures, such as writing a long introduction to introduce TCM and Huang Di Nei Jing, using appendixes and many footnotes in the translation to explain words and concepts unique in TCM and Chinese culture, thus providing essential cultural information for readers.

Today we know that Ilza Veith's translated version is full of errors, mistakes, and mistranslations due to less understanding TCM, archaic Chinese, etc. If its value is evaluated only from the aspect of language and the yardstick of "faithfulness", Ilza Veith's translation is of no value at all. But it is simply not the case. At that time, some authoritative medical journals such as Science, Archives of Internal Medicine, Journal of American Medical Association (JAMA), and California Medicine, highly appraised Ilza Veith's translated version of Nei Jing.

In the years of 1945-1949 when Ilza Veith translated the Nei Jing, in the West, Western medicine was in a self-sufficient state, and TCM therapies were mainly confined to descendants of Chinese or Asian although they had been transmitted to the West in the 17th century, and English translation of TCM works including ancient TCM classics was in a very marginal position in the Western medical cultural system; while in China, dissemination of Western medicine was catching on like fire throughout the country on one hand, position and role of TCM were in a all-time low on the other hand, disputation, interchange between and combination of TCM and Western medicine were becoming increasingly intense. Under such an outside environment, translation and publication of Huang Di Nei Jing in America at that time were of great opening significance.

It is worth to note that Ilza Veith's translation is still available today as time goes by. The back cover of the new edition of Ilza Veith's translation[1] wrote that "Since 1949, when the first translation of the oldest known document in Chinese medicine was published, traditional medical practice has been a dynamic revival in China. Moreover, it has spread amazingly through many countries of the Western world, even to the United States. Scientific investigations into the rationale of this time-honored therapy (including acupuncture) have heightened the interest in its historical and philosophical foundation. As Far Eastern thought and its history become increasingly more important factors in resent-day knowledge, The Yellow Emperor's Classic has gradually transcended the confines of medical history".

Since the establishment of the People's Republic of China in 1949, the Communist Party and government of China have attached great importance to development of TCM. In 1958, Chairman Mao Zedong wrote that "TCM is a great treasure house, which should be explored and improved with great efforts". In 1969, Primer Zhou Enlai pointed out in many speeches that "Doctors of Western medicine should learn from practitioners of TCM, which should be encouraged and become a common practice". Ren Min Ri Bao (People's Daily) announced achievement of success in acupuncture anesthesia on July 17th, 1971, which shocked the country and the whole world. "Acupuncture training courses for foreign doctors" were conducted in 1976 in Shanghai and Beijing. Soon afterwards, "International Acupuncture Training Centers" were set up in Beijing, Shanghai, and Nanjing with the help of WHO (World Health Organisation).

At a time like the present when Chinese medicine, particularly Chinese acupuncture therapy and anesthesia, is making its way into Western culture, the task of translating The Yellow Emperor's Books of Internal Medicine (Nei Jing) into English for the benefit of Western readers has, more than ever, become the necessity of the times.[2] A Complete Transla-

---

1   It was published by University of California Press, in 1972.
2   Henry C. Lu 1987, p.5

tion of Nei Jing and Nan Jing (Yellow Emperor's Classics) and The Yellow Emperor's Book of Acupuncture (containing a translation of the first 14 chapters of the Ling Shu and 3 supplements on the eight extraordinary meridians, modern application of meridians in acupuncture therapy and in acupuncture anesthesia) by Henry C. Lu were published by Academy of Oriental Heritage (USA and Canada) in 1978 and 1987 respectively. Dr. Henry C. Lu, Ph.D., as a multi-disciplinary student of an international background at that time and an English-speaking Chinese, took on the responsibility of "keeping Western readers in touch with the invaluable information contained in this first Chinese medical book, particularly in view of the fact that the book has proven to be a great deal more than just an ordinary book of medical history".[1]

Henry C. Lu classified the intended readers in his mind into the following three categories: "the students of Chinese history, medical or otherwise"; "the students of Chinese philosophy"; "all medical professionals who wish to practice Chinese medicine, acupuncture included".[2] It proves from another aspect that Henry C. Lu realized that the Nei Jing bears historical, philosophical, and medical values, and that he tried to contain and reproduce the three values in the translation.

Henry C. Lu translated the terminologies in TCM according to convention unless there were good reasons for translating them differently. For example, he followed the conventional translation of "五藏" and "六府", rendering them into "five viscera" and "six bowels" respectively; adopted "meridian" for Jing Mai 经脉, "energy" for Qi 气; translated Xin Bao 心包, which had been conventionally translated as "Circulatory Sex", as "Pericardium"; translated Du Mai 督脉, which had been conventionally translated as "Governing Vessel", as "Axis Meridian"; adopted some Western medical terms to translate TCM concepts, such as "rheumatism" for Bi 痹. It shows that Henry C. Lu adopted a combined translation strategy of "foreignization" and "domestication".

As regards to interpretation and translation of the original text, Henry C. Lu said in Translator's Explanatory Remarks, "There exist some basic agreements among the Chinese acupuncturists regarding the interpretation of the original text. In case of ambiguities, however, the following two

---

1   Henry C. Lu 1987, p.5
2   Ibid.

principles are followed in translating them: one, the principle of consistency throughout the text; two, conformity to the modern theory of Chinese acupuncture".

We can see from his choice of translation strategy and principles that he laid special emphasis on acceptability of the translation to the intended readers, stressing conveying TCM knowledge, translating and introducing the Nei Jing to Western readers as an "authoritative reference" of TCM.

A Proposed Standard International Acupuncture Nomenclature appraised and approved by WHO came out in 1991 in Geneva. Maoshing Ni's translation of the Nei Jing Su Wen was published by Shambhala (Boston and London) in 1995.

Ni, Maoshing, Ph.D., D.O.M., was born and raised in a family medical tradition that spans many generations, and is an author, lecturer, and licensed practitioner of TCM in the United States. Dr. Ni studied TCM with his father, a renowned physician and author, and also received advanced training in China and the United States. Dr. Ni has compiled, translated, and published several books on TCM in The United States. In A Note on the Translation of translated version of Huang Di Nei Jing Su Wen, he said, "This translation, however, was never meant to be a scholarly edition. For that purpose I am certain that other improvements can be made by expert sinologists. Instead, I have approached this from a clinician's point of view, all the while keeping in mind the criteria of students of traditional Chinese medicine and philosophy as well as those of interested laypersons".[1]

It is thus clear that the translator, as a practitioner of TCM (his cultural status), with students of TCM and philosophy as well as those of interested laypersons as intended readers, translated and interpreted Huang Di Nei Jing Su Wen in a light and popular style, laying special emphasis on introducing TCM knowledge in the book. At the same time, he admitted his deficiency in philology (understanding the original text), and affirmed that a better translation will come out with the help of expert sinologist in the future. Actually, we can regard Ni's translated version as a modern interpretation of Huang Di Nei Jing Su Wen in English.

At Ni's time, TCM has been disseminated to the world over at an unprecedented speed, esp. in the United States; and TCM has been gradu-

---

1   Maoshing Ni 1995, p.XIV

ally entering the medical system of English speaking countries. English translation of TCM works has been gradually moving to the center of the medical cultural poly-system of the English speaking countries. Western readers' interest in TCM is steadily on the increase, and their acceptability to TCM is growing stronger and stronger with each passing day. The outside environment enables Ni to adopt "foreignization" as the main translation strategy to express unique TCM concepts, and not use Western medical terms indiscriminately. His translation accords with the developing tendency of English translation of TCM. For example, Dr. Ni adopted "channels" (a popular translation in the West for "经脉"), or "meridians" (a standardized translation for "经脉" approved by WHO) for "经脉"; adopted the method of pinyin transliteration + explanation to translate "天癸" into "tian kui, or fertility essence"; calmly rendered "脾" into "spleen", "肾" into "kidney" when facing the great difference of the function of the spleen and kidneys between TCM and Western medicine. Moreover, Dr. Ni did not introduce TCM or Huang Di Nei Jing in a separate space or use footnotes for the cause of publication of English TCM works has been flourishing in the West, and his translation is very fluent in language.

Paul Unschuld is a medical historian. He did not mention his cultural status (medical historian? sinologist? or practitioner of TCM?) like Ilza Veith or Dr. Ni in the first publication---Huang Di Nei Jing Su Wen: Nature, Knowledge, Imagery in An Ancient Chinese Medical Text of the Su Wen project when translating Su Wen. In the Prefatory Remarks of the first publication, he expressed the following ideas: (1) The Huang Di nei jing su wen plays a major role in Chinese medical history comparable to that of the Hippocratic writings in ancient Europe. (2) Up till now, many practitioners of Chinese medicine still consider the Su Wen a valuable source of theoretical inspiration and practical knowledge in modern clinical settings. (3) Reading the Su Wen can increase our understanding of the roots of Chinese medicine as an integral aspect of Chinese civilisation, help judge the poly-system of medical culture where TCM and Western medicine co-exist, and provide a much needed starting point for serious and well-informed discussions on the topic. (4) The final translation is the result of nearly 20 years of international cooperation with philologist and expert in TCM. Thus it can be seen that Unschuld lays equal stress on medical knowledge, historical value, and philological aspect, and tries to comprehensively reproduce the values of Huang Di Nei Jing Su Wen in the translation. Such a translation approach is closely related to the remarkable promotion of TCM in the poly-system of medical culture of the English speaking countries, esp. the USA.

During the 19 years when Unschuld devoted himself to the translation of Huang Di Nei Jing Su Wen, legislation, education, and publication on TCM, on acumoxatherapy in particular, have been developing very rapidly in the United States. The Final Report of the White House Commission on Complementary and Alternative Medicine Policy came out in March of 2002. Therapies of TCM and acupuncture are not "folk therapies" anymore, and have gained "legal status and position". Under such a social background, as regards to the translation strategy, Unschuld did not hesitate to break free from conventions and conventional standards of TCM translation of the English speaking countries, making English TCM terminology in the translation having a unique system of his own for the purpose of making the translation near the original in the aspect of "adequacy" (i.e. main textual relationship of the reproduction of the original) as possible as he can. He has suggested a rational criterion for determining whether a metaphor is alive or dead. He argues that since TCM claims to follow the conceptual system laid down in the Nei Jing, metaphors that were alive when the Nei Jing was written should be carried over in translation.[1] For example, he rendered "藏府" into "depots and palaces", "经脉" into "conduit vessel" (i.e. "conduit" for"经", "vessel" for"脉"), "经络学说" into "The Vessel Theory", "五行学说" into "The Five-Agents Doctrine" (He followed Harper and Marc Kalinowski's suggestion to translate wu xing as "five agents"), and so and so forth.

In the Prefatory Remarks, Unschuld said, "This book cannot and does not claim to say everything that can be said about the Su Wen. On the contrary, it should be seen merely as a beginning, meant to generate an intellectual interest in this text in many more scholars than have cared to take notice of it and related ancient Chinese writings in the past".[2] It shows that the translators' aim of translation is to generate an intellectual interest in this text and other TCM ancient texts in many more scholars and his intended readers are not popular people but scholars of related

---

1 Nigel Wiseman 1996, p.63
2 Unschuld 2003, XII

academic fields. We can regard Unschuld's translation as the first complete translation in a scholar sense.

For the purpose of making readers or scholars truly enjoy reading and understanding Huang Di Nei Jing Su Wen, Unschuld adopted many compensatory measures: The first publication *Huang Di Nei Jing Su Wen: Nature, Knowledge, Imagery in An Ancient Chinese Medical Text* gives the Su Wen a comprehensive and deep-going introduction, and involves a comparative study of early medical history of the West and the related part of the Su Wen; In the forthcoming translation, besides the translation, he also selectively translated reasonable annotations and explanations from more than six hundred related monographs; Hermann Tessenow has conducted a detailed analysis of the approximately three hundred fifty separate segments constituting the historical and structural layers of the Su Wen (several volumes).

It is thus clear that translator's awareness of medical culture of the target language and awareness of intended readers are influenced by translator's cultural status and intention, and his or her outside environment, thus manifesting in his or her choice of translation strategy, the purpose of translation, and concrete translating methods. The phenomena of "creative treason" in the translation are the breakthrough point of the research on translator's awareness of medical culture of the target language and awareness of the intended readers.

3. The Required Accomplishments of the Nei Jing translator

The same literary works usually has different and independent aesthetic quality and style in different translator's eyes. Huang Di Nei Jing is not a literary works, so its translation is different from translation of literary works. Translation of Nei Jing can be regarded as translation of classical works and translation of scientific and technological works. Translator should translate Nei Jing according to his or her capacity if he or she wants to translate it. Here, "capacity" refers to various factors which influence or even determine the translator to bring his or her subjectivities into full and good play.

All the Chinese medical classics, including Nei Jing, bear historical, medical, and cultural values. If the translator is a medical historian, he will stress the historical value of the works; if the translator is a practitioner of TCM, he or she will stress the medical value of the classic, trying to express the medical knowledge contained in the classic; if the translator is a sinologist or a philologist, he or she will stress the cultural or philological aspect of the classic. But anyway, no matter who the translator is, if he or she wants to translate Huang Di Nei Jing, he or she should satisfy the following requirements:

(1) Possessing some knowledge of biliology, exegetics, and textual criticism of ancient TCM documents for the purpose of selecting a good edition as the original, reading, understanding, and distinguishing related annotations, commentaries of the text made through the past ages.

(2) Possessing TCM academic background and reading comprehension of archaic Chinese for the purpose of reading, understanding, and interpreting the original text of the Huang Di Nei Jing with the aid of dictionaries and annotations of the past ages, then translate the original text not the modern Chinese interpretations into English. (Up till now, only Ilza Veith and Paul Unschuld directly translated the original text not the modern Chinese interpretation.)

(3) Having a good grounding in basic skills of the target language (English) and translation accomplishment for the purpose of reproducing the ideas, contents, linguistic style of the Huang Di Nei Jing with the target language (English).

(4) Being aware of medical culture of the target language (English), being familiar with the position and practical significance of TCM and Huang Di Nei Jing in the poly-system of the medical culture of the target language (English), clarifying the translation objective, for the purpose of adopting corresponding translation strategy and concrete translation methods and avoiding translating behind the closed doors by divorcing himself or herself from the social reality without any aim.

(5) Being aware of the intended readers, clarifying "translating for whom", for the purpose of attracting the intended readers in mind by adopting all rational methods and measures at any moment in the whole translating process.

4. Who Possess the Required Accomplishments of Nei Jing Translation and How to Translate It?

But who possess the above mentioned requirements? Actually, there is no single person who possesses all of the requirements. The only solution is to organize personnel in related specific fields of China and target language country to translate a particular classic through international cooperation.

The thesis points out that only after making a thorough investigation and a thorough study on the classic text to be translated the translators can begin the actual translating work. It also emphasizes that the translation should embody the close combination of translation and study as an essential condition.

For a scholarly translation, to be more specific, the translators should observe the following procedures:

(1) Organize personnel in related specific fields of China and target language country to translate a particular classic,

(2) choose a reliable text as the source text,

(3) choose and follow what is good about the existing critical commentaries and various annotations made throughout the ages on the text,

(4) proceed to translate the source text, making sure to include the specific terminology, all the sentences and different sections as well as the metaphors those may contain, adopting as much as possible, a word-to-word literal approach so as to reproduce the content, form, and style of the source text in an English version that is completely faithful to the original,

(5) select and adopt various measures that may help to comprehensively and thoroughly introduce the cultural connotations of the classic text, making the final translation work reflect the process of Chinese learning within the Chinese medical context,

(6) compile the indexes of the Chinese & English versions of this particular classic.

All the Chinese medical classics, including Nei Jing, bear a combination of historical, medical, and cultural values. Translating Chinese medical classics in accordance with the above-mentioned procedures would make these historical medical, and cultural values also appear in their English versions. Such an approach would, therefore, also make it possible for the Western readers to completely understand the Chinese medical and cultural heritage and for traditional Chinese medicine to be better known, studied and appreciated world-wide with a brighter future for many years to come.

Acknowledgement: I am very grateful to Nicole Command and Dr. G. Kubiena for providing me invaluable materials which are indispensable to the accomplishment of the thesis.

Table: Brief Introduction to Translations of *Huangdi's Inner Classic*

	Year Published	Translator	Title of the Translation	Content of the Translation	Length of Translation	Additional Parts
1	1925	Dawson, Percy. M. M.D.	Su-wen, the Basis of Chinese Medicine	Abridged translation of *Su Wen*	6 pages	/
2	1949	Veith, Ilza Ph. D. in History of Medicine	The Yellow Emperor's Classic of Internal Medicine	Chapters 1-34 of *Su We*	32K, totally 260 pages, translation: 156 pages	Prefaces, Introduction to *Nei Jing* (76 page), Appendix 1-3. Bibliography, and Translation
3	1950	Huang Wen Doctor, President of Sun Yixian Medical School	Nei Ching, the Chinese Canon of Medicine	Translation of important chapters and sections of *Su Wen* and commentaries	33 pages	/
4	1978	Lu, Henry C. Ph.D., Practitioner of TCM in Canada	A Complete Translation of *Nei Jing and Nan Jing* (Yellow Emperor's Classics)	A complete translation of *Nei Jing and Nan Jing*	Unknown	Unknown
5	1987	Lu, Henry C. Ph.D., Practitioner of TCM in Canada	The Yellow Emperor's Book of Acupuncture	Chapters 1-14 of *Ling Shu*	257 pages	3 Supplements on the eight extraordinary meridians, modern application of meridians in acupuncture therapy and in acupuncture anesthesia

No.	Year	Translator	Title	Description	Size	Notes
6	1995	Ni, Maoshing Ph.D., M.D., Practitioner of TCM in the USA	The Yellow Emperor's Classic of Medicine: A New Translation of the *Nei Jing Su Wen* with Commentary	A complete translation of *Su Wen* with commentary	32K, 301 pages	Prefaces, Bibliography, About the Translator, Index, etc.
7	1997	Unsigned	The Illustrated Yellow Emperor's Canon of Medicine	Selected translation of chapters and sections involving health preservation with cartoon and typical examples	16K, 209 pages	13 medicinal recipes from *Nei Jing* and Nourishing Your True Nature
8	Dec., 1997	Wu, Lianheng; Wu, Qi Practitioners (father-son) of TCM in the USA	The Yellow Emperor's Canon Internal Medicine	A complete translation of *Nei Jing* (Chinese-English)	16K, 831 pages	/
9	2001	Zhu Ming Practitioner of TCM in China	The Medical Classic of the Yellow Emperor	The 5th ed. of the *Textbook of Nei Jing* for TCM Higher Education	32K, 302 pages	Unknown
10	June, 2002	Wu Jing-Nuan founder of the Taoist Health Institute	Ling Shu, The Spiritual Pivot	A complete Translation of *Ling Shu*	283 pages	/
11	2003	Unschuld, Paul U; Tessenau, Hermann; Zheng Jinsheng Professors of History of Medicine; Philologist	HUANG DI NEI JING SU WEN	A complete translation of *Su Wen* after consulting over 3000 related theses and commentaries of over 600 related works of the past ages, and other achievements	Translation: 3 volumes, still not published	*HUANG DI NEI JING SU WEN: Nature, Knowledge, Imagery in An Ancient Chinese Medical Text* (2003); *Dictionary of the Huangdi Neijing Suwen* (2007)

101

References

Editorial Department of Chinese Translators Journal 1992, *Collected Works of Skills in Chinese-English Translating* [C], Beijing: China Translation & Publishing Corporation.

Guo Aichun 1999, *Collation, Annotation and Modern Translation of Huang Di Nei Jing Su Wen*,Tianjin: Tianjin Science and Technology Press.

Huang Wen. Nei Ching 1950, the Chinese Canon of Medicine [J], *Chinese Medical Journal*, 68:1-2.

Ji Wenhui, Wang Damei 2000, *Bibliology of Ancient Chinese Medical Documents* [M], Shanghai: Shanghai Scientific and Technical Publishers.

Lan Fengli 2004, Discussion on the English Translation of the Book Name of Huang Di Nei Jing Su Wen, *Chinese Journal of Integrated Traditional and Western Medicine*, (2):175-177.

Lan Fengli 2004, On English Translation of Titles of Sections in Huang Di Nei Jing Su Wen, *Chinese Journal of Integrated Traditional and Western Medicine*,(3): 265-268.

Lan Fengli 2004, A Descriptive Study of the English Translation of Huang Di Nei Jing Su Wen (1) [J], *Chinese Journal of Integrated Traditional and Western Medicine*, (10): 947-950.

Lan Fengli 2005, A Descriptive Study of the English Translation of Huang Di Nei Jing Su Wen (2) [J], *Chinese Journal of Integrated Traditional and Western Medicine*, (2):176-180.

Lan Fengli 2005. *Cultural Connotations and Translation of Ancient Chinese Medical Classics*. Ph.D. Dissertation. Shanghai University of Traditional Chinese Medicine.

Lu Yuling 2004, The Spirit of Translation: A Comment on Who Translates? Translator Subjectivities Beyond Reason by Douglas Robinson, *Chinese Translator's Journal*, (2): 56.

Lu, Henry C 1987, *The Yellow Emperor's Book of Acupuncture,* Vancouver: Academy of Oriental Heritage.

Nelson Liansheng Wu, Andrew Qi Wu 1997, *Yellow Empero's Canon Internal Medicine*, Beijing: China Science & Technology Press.

Ni, Maoshing 1995, The *Yellow Emperor's Classic of Medicine*, Boston, Massachusetts: Shambhala.

Robinson, Douglas 2001, *Who Translates? Translator Subjectivities Beyond Reason* [M], New York: State University of New York Press.

Translators Zhou Ning, Jin Yuanpu 1987, *Receptive Aesthetics and Receptive Theory*,Shenyang: Liaoning People's Publishing House.

Unschuld, Paul U 2003, *HUANG DI NEI JING SU WEN: Nature, Knowledge, Imagery in An Ancient Chinese Medical Text* [M], Berkeley, Los Angeles and London: University of California Press, IX-XII.

Veith,Ilza 1972, *The Yellow Emperor's Classic of Internal Medicine*. New ed., Berkeley, Los Angeles and London: University of California Press.

Wang Chimin 1936, Re-investigation into Translation of Chinese Medical Classics into Western Languages [J], *Chinese Medical Journal* (Chinese Version), 22 (12): 1229-1234.

Wang Chimin, Fu Weikang 1966, *Index of the Literature in Foreign Languages on History of Chinese Medicine (1682-1965)* [M], Shanghai: Museum of Chinese Medical History of Shanghai College of Traditional Chinese Medicine.

Wang Zuoliang 1989, *Translation, Experiments and Reflections*,Beijing: Foreign Language Teaching and Research Press.

Wiseman, Nigel 1996, English-Chinese Chinese-English Dictionary of Chinese Medicine,Hunan Science & Technology Press, 22.

Xu Jun 2003, Creative Treason and the Establishment of Translational Subjectivity [J], *Chinese Translators Journal*, (1): 11.

Zha Mingjian, Tian Yu 2003, On the Subjectivity of the Translator [J], *Chinese Translators Journal*, (1): 22.

Zhou Chuncai, Han Yazhou 1997, *The Illustrated Yellow Emperor's Canon of Medicine (Chinese-English)*, Beijing: Dolphin Books.

Zhu Ming 2001, *The Medical Classic of the Yellow Emperor* [M], Beijing: Foreign Languages Press.

Lan Fengli

The Origin and Translation of Qi, Yin-Yang and Wu Xing in TCM

Qi, Yin-Yang, and Wu Xing are originally concepts in the classical Chinese philosophy. On the basis of long-term medical practice, ancient Chinese medical experts introduced them into TCM, and applied them extensively to the medical field to explain origin of the life, physiological functions and pathological changes of the human being, and to guide diagnosis, prevention and treatment of diseases in clinical practice. Thus, they have become vital component parts of the fundamental theories of TCM, and have deeply influenced the formation and development of the theoretical system of TCM.

1. The Origin and Translation of "Qi" in TCM

The Origin of Chinese Characters • Qi Part (Shuo Wen Jie Zi •Qi Bu, 《说文解字•气部》) states that "Qi refers to thin, floating clouds. The character 气 is a pictographic character." The character 气 in Jia Gu Wen, the inscriptions on bones or tortoise shells of the Shang Dynasty (c. 16th-11th century B.C.), was written as "川", which resembles air current, evaporating and rising, whose image is just like cloud, will disappear very soon and become invisible. Therefore, qi is invisible and formless, exists everywhere, can be gathered into a form, for instance, qi can be condensed into water. Qi at this moment can be translated into air or vapor.

Soon afterwards, the qi which surrounds and congests the space of the human being was abstracted into the qi which bears a material meaning in philosophical sense. Philosophers of materialism of the Spring Autumn and Warring States Period (770-221B.C.) believed that qi is the basic material constituting the world, and that everything in the universe comes into being by the movement and mutation of qi. For example, Book of Changes • Section Xi Ci, (Zhou Yi •Xi Ci, 《周易•系辞》), states that "everything is transformed and generated by the enshrouding [qi] of the heaven and earth".

Later on, ancient Chinese medical experts introduced "qi" into the medical field at the right moment. And then, "qi" became a medium or bridge between the natural philosophy of the pre-Qin days (i.e. before 221 B.C. when the First Emperor of Qin united China) and Chinese medicine. The concept of "qi" gradually formed in TCM.

In the time of Huangdi's Inner Classic, "qi" is regarded not only as the basic material constituting the world, but also as the basic material constituting the human being which can be transformed into blood, essence, and body fluid, etc., and the normal functional activities of the life which is governed by "qi" is known as Shen or spirit. For example, Plain Questions • Discourse on Protecting Life and Preserving Physical Appearance (Su Wen • Baoming Quanxing Lun, 《素问•宝命全形论》) states that "The human being is generated by qi of the heaven and earth, and is completed by the law of the four seasons"; And that "the union of qi of the heaven and earth gives birth to the human being". Actually, there are abundant accounts of qi in the Plain Questions. Only the monosyllabic word "qi" appears 1176 times in Plain Questions. Almost all the 79 existing chapters of the Plain Questions discuss qi. All the theories and skills of the Plain Questions are related to qi. And there are various qi with a multitude of names in the Plain Questions, such as yin qi, yang qi; clear qi, turbid qi; heaven qi, earth qi; right qi or healthy qi, evil qi or pathogenic qi; nutritive qi, defensive qi; seasonal qi, visceral qi, meridian qi; and so and so forth (see Lan Fengli 2006, pp.201-05).

According to A Concise Dictionary of Chinese Medicine (Jian Ming Zhong Yi Ci Dian, 《简明中医词典》), qi in TCM bears the following meanings: (1) nutritious, essential substance flowing inside the body, such as food qi, breathed air, (2) functional activities of the zang-fu organs in a general sense, such as visceral qi (i.e, the functional activities of the zang-fu organs); qi can also be classified into original qi, nutritive qi, defensive qi, pectoral qi, etc. according to its source, distribution, and function, (3) the location or stage of pattern identification of warm diseases (see Li Jingwei 2001, p.173).

It is thus clear that qi was not air or vapor long ago. And then, what is qi in TCM? Energy? Vital energy? Atmosphere? Or influence? For qi implies many meanings and any translation can not convey all the cultural connotations of qi, and therefore, I believe pinyin transliteration is the best choice for qi. But more important, the presupposition of pinyin transliteration is that you should know the origin, development and cultural connotations of qi.

2. The Origin and Translation of "Yin-Yang" in TCM

Yin-yang is a pair of concepts in the classical Chinese philosophy. The original meanings of yin-yang are very simple and plain, i.e. the side facing the sun being yang and the reverse side being yin. Later on, yin-yang has by extension come to mean cold-hot of the weather, upwards-downwards, right-left, and inwards-outwards of the directions, excitement-quiescence and motion-motionlessness of the moving states, and so and so forth. In the classical TCM texts, yin-yang bears rich and varied meanings. Since the specific meanings of yin and yang depend highly upon the linguistic context in which they appear, it is ill-advised to consistently use their pinyin transliterations in rendering the two concepts into other languages. To be adequate, their translation should accord with the actual contextual meanings they have acquired.

2.1 The Origin of "Yin-Yang" in TCM

It was Bo Yang Fu (伯阳父) of the last years of Western Zhou Dynasty (C. 1100-771B.C.) that first used the word yin-yang, gave it the abstract meaning of opposition, and used it to explain natural phenomena. He believed that "yang hides [inside] and can not come out, yin is forced and can not ascend, and then earthquake ensues" (Guo Yu •Zhou Yu, 《国语·周语》). Fan Li (范蠡) of the last years of Spring-Autumn Period (770-476B.C.) said that "yang in its extreme becomes yin, and yin in its extreme becomes yang; the sun in the end rises again, and the moon in the full wanes" (Guo Yu •Yue Yu, 《国语· 越语》), which was the first and earliest formulation of waxing-waning and transformation of yin-yang. Lao Zi • 42nd Chapter (《老子·四十二章》) states that "everything in the universe bears yin and embraces yang, where the central and harmonious qi makes them in harmony". This quotation affirms that the contradictory qualities of yin-yang are intrinsic attributes of everything.

106

Book of Changes (Yi Zhuan, 《易传》) further advances that "one yin and one yang makes Tao", which abstracts yin-yang to the extensive universality and regards yin-yang as the fundamental rule of the universe for the first time. Book of Changes also uses yin-yang to make a comparison of social phenomena, and yin-yang has by extension come to imply the relationship between upward and downward, monarch and ministers, wife and husband, etc. Joseph Needham believed that yin-yang as definite philosophical term appears in the Book of Changes. Dong Zhongshu's Chun Qiu Fan Lu (董仲舒《春秋繁露》) states that "the heaven has yin-yang, the human being also has yin-yang. Yin qi of the heaven rises and yin qi of the human being will respond it to rise, while yin qi of the human being rises and yin qi of the heaven will respond it to rise too. The principles or ways are the same".

TCM inherits and develops the idea of yin-yang in the Book of Changes. For example, Plain Questions• Great Discourse on Images Corresponding to Yin-Yang (Su Wen • Yin-Yang Ying Xiang Da Lun, 《素问•阴阳应象大论》) states that

"Yin and yang, they are
the Way of heaven and earth,
the fundamental principles [governing] the myriad being,
father and mother to all changes and transformations,
the basis and beginning of generating and killing,
the palace of spirit brilliance."[1]

To the human being, yin-yang is the supreme headquarters of the mental activities.

Not all of the yin-yang in ancient medical texts is abstract philosophical concept. For example, among the medical books unearthed in the Mawangdui Han Tomb (马王堆汉墓), Ten Questions (Shi Wen 《十问》) discusses the way of meeting yin [the female's genitals]; Methods of Integrating Yin and Yang (He Yin-Yang Fang 《合阴阳方》) on the methods of copulation of the male and female; Supreme Way of the Land under Heaven (Tian Xia Zhi Dao Tan 《天下至道谈》) on harms and benefits of sexual intercourse; Way of Preserving Health (Yang Sheng Fang 《养生方》) and Miscellaneous Therapies (Za Liao Fang 《杂疗方》) on function

---

1   Unschuld 2003, p.86

of sexual intercourse and antenatal instruction. The theory of yin-yang is easy to tally with the male and female in the sexual intercourse. So, it is very natural to use the principles of yin-yang to explain the sexual intercourse or even use yin-yang as a synonym or euphemism of the sexual intercourse in the above-mentioned works. These works on sexual intercourse press close to the philosophy of yin-yang on one end and to the medical life on the other. So yin-yang can be regarded as a bridge between philosophy and medicine. Thus, it is very common in ancient Chinese medical texts to adopt yin-yang to represent male and female and sexual intercourse as in the Mawangdui medical books.

Moreover, ancient Chinese medical classics applied yin-yang theory extensively into the medical field. Take the Plain Questions (Su Wen) as an Example. There are 45 chapters discussing yin-yang in the existing 79 chapters of the book, which proves that the relationship between yin-yang and medicine is vitally important.

In the Book of Changes, yin-yang is mainly used in the field of natural philosophy; while in TCM, yin-yang is used not only in philosophical field, but also in medical field, and yin-yang is an ingenious unification of philosophical and medical senses. Huangdi's inner Classic (Huang Di Nei Jing, 《黄帝内经》) makes a more systematic and definite expression on the ideas of interdependence, waning-waxing, transformation, harmony of yin-yang implied in the Book of Changes, develops these ideas in combination with medical practice, and makes yin-yang theory become the guiding theory of TCM.

In a word, TCM inherits and develops the idea of yin-yang in the Book of Changes. Yin-yang in Ancient Chinese medical texts mainly refers to philosophical yin-yang. But yin-yang in concrete medical texts may refer to some specific medical meanings, such as the male and female, sex or sexual activity, yin-yang meridians, yin-yang pathogens, yin-yang qi, etc. The meaning of "阴阳" depends highly upon the language context.

2.2 Translation of "Yin-Yang" in TCM

2.2.1 Translation of "Yin-Yang" in Philosophical Sense

There is no way of investigating when "yin-yang" concepts were transmitted into the West. Let's take a look at how Ilza Veith translated "yin-yang" in Huangdi' s Inner Classic in the 1940s:

"Yin and Yang [the male and female elements in nature];
Yang, the element of light; Yin, the element of darkness;
Yin and Yang, the negative and positive principles in nature;
The element of light; the element of darkness;
Yang, the lucid element of life; Yin, the turbid element of darkness;
Yang, the male element; Yin, the female element;
Yin and Yang [the two elements in nature];
Yang, the lucid element; Yin, the turbid element;
Yin and Yang [the two opposing principles];
Yang (the male principle of light and life);
Yin (the female principle of darkness and death);...[1]"

It is thus clear that the Western people did not fully understand the meaning of "yin-yang" at the Veith's time: yin-yang was occasionally translated into the element of light and the element of darkness; in most cases, yin-yang was pinyin transliterated with a concrete explanation. Actually, yin-yang has already gone beyond concrete meanings and has become philosophical concept with broad and abstract senses.

As we all know, yin and yang have been included in English dictionaries, such as Longman Dictionary of Contemporary English: "yin, the female principle in Chinese PHILOSOPHY which is inactive, dark, negative, etc. and which combines with YANG (= the male principle) to form the whole world"; "yang, the male principle in Chinese PHILOSOPHY which is active, light, POSITIVE, etc. and which combines with YIN (= the female principle) to form the whole world".[2] While Webster's Encyclopedic Unabridged Dictionary of the English Language combines yin and yang into one item: "Yin and Yang (in Chinese philosophy and religion) two principles, one negative, dark and feminine (Yin), and one positive, bright, and masculine (Yang), whose interaction influences the destinies of creatures and things."[3]

Thus it can be seen that "yin" was originally translated into the female, negative, inactive, dark, or turbid principle or element, and "yang" was

1   Veith 1949, pp.97-253
2   Longman Dictionary of Contemporary English: 1789, 1787; 1998
3   Webster's Encyclopedic Unabridged Dictionary of the English Language: 1656, 1994

originally translated into the male, positive, active, bright, or lucid principle or element in the West. As time went by, the Westerners came to find that whatever word(s) could not cover all the philosophical meanings implied in "yin-yang", finally accepted the two loan words: yin and yang.

Actually, yin-yang can also help express other particular terms of TCM for yin-yang has been accepted by the English language. For example, wu zang (五脏) pertains to yin, liu fu (六腑 pertains to yang. So wu zang can be translated into "the (five) yin organs", liu fu can be translated into "the (six) yang organs" (see Kaptchuk 2000, pp.75-95), which are apparently more acceptable to the Western readers than "the five zang organs and" and "the six fu organs" (see Xie Zhufan 2002, p.14). But I believe that "the five zang organs and" and "the six fu organs" will be finally accepted by the Westerners with further transmission of TCM to the West.

2.2.2 Translation of "Yin-Yang" as Concrete Concept

The meaning of yin-yang varies with the concrete language context. Yin-yang may refer to such concrete concepts as female and male, sexual activity, yin meridians and yang meridians, yin qi and yang qi, etc. When yin-yang is used as concrete concept, yin-yang should be translated into their corresponding specific meanings.

A. Original Text: 《素问·上古天真论》：丈夫八岁，肾气实，发长齿更；二八，肾气盛，天癸至，精气溢泻，阴阳和，故能有子。

Translation: In the male, at the age of eight the boy's kidney qi is abundant, his hair grows and his baby teeth are replaced by permanent ones. At the age of 16 the tian gui or sex-stimulating essence matures, he begins to secrete semen; if at this point the male and female unite in harmony, a child may be conceived.

Notes: Here, "yin-yang" refers to female and male. "实" should be "盛". "肾气盛" is redundancy. "和" should be "和合", i.e. unite in harmony (see Guo Aichun 1999, p.4).

B. Original Text: 《诸病源候论·妇人杂病诸候·带下候》：冲任之脉既起于胞内，阴阳过度，则伤胞络，故风邪乘虚而入于胞，损冲、任之经，伤太阳、少阴之血，致令胞络之间，秽液与血相兼，连带而下。

Translation: The conception (or controlling) and thoroughfare vessels both originate from the uterus. Excessive sexual activities harms uterine collaterals, and then pathogenic wind invades the uterus, impairing the two vessels, damaging blood of Taiyang and Shaoyin, causing turbidity and blood in the uterine collaterals, together with vaginal discharge, flowing down out of the body.

Notes: Here, "yin-yang" refers to sexual activity.

C. Original Text: 《灵枢·口问》：百病之始生也，皆生于风雨寒暑、阴阳喜怒、饮食居处、大惊卒恐。

Translation: Various diseases are caused by exposure to wind, rain, cold or summer-heat, or excess sex, or a lack of harmonious emotions, or improper diet, or a lack of regularity in lifestyle, or great fear or sudden fright.

Notes: Here, "yin-yang" refers to excessive sexual activities or excess sex.

D. Original Text: 《素问·疏五过论》：粗工治之，亟刺阴阳，身体解散，四支转筋，死日有期。

Translation: A careless doctor treats it by pricking the yin and yang meridians time and again, thus causing the patient getting emaciated, having crumps in the limbs and coming closer to the death day.

Notes: Here, "yin-yang" refers to yin meridians and yang meridians. The standardized translation for "经脉" approved by WHO (World Health Organisation) is meridian (a two-dimensional grid). Seeing that "经脉" can carry and move qi and blood and must be a three-dimensional tube, channel indicating a three-dimensional tube also become a very popular translation for "经脉".

E. Original Text: 《素问·调经论》：夫阴与阳，皆有俞会，阳注于阴，阴满之外，阴阳匀平，以充其形，九候若一，命曰平人。夫邪之生也，或生于阴，或生于阳，其生于阳者，得之风雨寒暑；其生于阴者，得之饮食居处、阴阳喜怒。

Translation: The yin and yang meridians possess acupuncture points, where transportation and convergence of qi and blood occur. Blood and qi of the yang meridians will transport to the yin meridians. Blood and qi then fill the yin meridians and flow to other parts of the body. Then yin and yang are balanced, the body becomes robust, the nine indicators of the body's pulses will also be concert. This occurs in a normal, healthy person. The pathogens may attack the body. There are internal damages caused by yin pathogens and external contractions caused by yang pathogens. The external contractions caused by yang pathogens may result from exposure to rain, wind, cold, or summer heat; while the internal damages caused by yin pathogens may arise from improper diet, a lack of regularity in lifestyle, excessive sexual activities, or a lack of harmonious emotions.

Notes: "Yin and yang" in "夫阴与阳" refers to the yin and yang meridians; "yin-yang" in "阴阳匀平" refers to abstract yin-yang, thus should be pinyin transliterated into yin and yang; as to "yin and yang" in "或生于阴，或生于阳", Zhang Qi (张琦) said that "there are internal damages caused by yin pathogens, and there are external contractions caused by yang pathogens"; "yin-yang" in "阴阳喜怒" refers to female and male, sexual activity, here refers to excessive sexual activities. Undoubtedly, such explanation is correct in view of medical principles (see Guo Aichun 1999, p.339).

F. Original Text: 《神农本草经卷三·中品》：蘗木，味苦，寒。主治五脏、肠胃中结热；黄疸；肠痔；止泄痢；女子漏下赤白；阴阳伤；蚀疮。

Translation: Phellodendri Cortex (Huang Bai), bitter in flavor and cold in property. Indications: accumulated heat in the five zang organs, the stomach and intestines; jaundice; perianal abscess; arresting diarrhea and dysentery; spotting with red or light-colored discharge in women; hypersexuality; sores resistant to healing.

Notes: Here, "yin-yang" refers to female's and male's genitals. "伤" is interchangeable with "壮". Yin-yang shang (阴阳伤) refers to exuberant sexual desire of female's and male's genitals, i.e. female and male having strong lust for sex, i.e. hypersexuality. In the quotation "望卿走，自投井死，昭信出之，椓杙其阴中" from Han Shu, the Historical Book of Han Dynasty(《汉书·景十三王传·广川惠王刘越》), yin refers to the female's genitals; in the quotation "囝生南方，闽吏得之乃绝其阳" from Nan, Boys, by Gu Kuang of the Tang Dynasty (唐·顾况《囝》), yang refers to the boy's genitals. Guang Ya, (《广雅·释诂四》), states that " 壮 is 伤". In the quotation "带甲婴马害歌於行伍，使人身伤" from Xun Zi(《荀子·乐论》), Yu Xinwu,(于新吾) explains that "伤 should be read as 壮" (see Gu Guangguang,Yang Pengju 2002, pp.175-76).

G. Original Text:《难经·五十八难》：伤寒之脉，阴阳俱盛而紧涩；热病之脉，阴阳俱浮，浮之而滑，沉之散涩。

Translation: The pulse of cold damage: both cun and chi pulses are strong, tense, and choppy. The pulse of febrile disease: both cun and chi pulses are floating; the pulses are slippery when felt slightly, and scattered and choppy when felt heavily.

Notes: Here, "yin-yang" refers to chi portion and cun portion of the pulse respectively for chi pertains to yin and cun pertains to yang.

H Original Text: 《伤寒论》：阴阳相搏，名曰动。阳动则汗出，阴动则发热。

Translation: When yin qi and yang qi wrestle with each other, the pulse is throbbing. When the cun pulse is throbbing, sweating results; when the chi pulse is throbbing, fever ensues.

Notes: "Yin-yang" in "阴阳相搏" refers to yin qi and yang qi; "yang" in "阳动"refers to the cun pulse, and "yin" in "阴动" refers to the chi pulse (see Li Peisheng, Cheng Zhaoren 2006, p.613).

Undoubtedly, ancient Chinese medical texts are vital original texts to study TCM. In the modern society, most of the readers of these ancient texts are practitioners of TCM who want to draw on TCM knowledge of the texts and apply the knowledge to clinical practice. So I advocate that translators should choose and follow what is good about the existing critical commentaries and various annotations made through the ages on the texts to make the translation reflect a generally recognised reasonable explanation; and that "yin-yang" can not all be pinyin transliterated, its translation should be determined by its concrete and specific meanings in the different contexts.

3. The Origin and Translation of "Wu Xing" in TCM
3.1 The Origin of "Wu Xing" in TCM

In fact, wu xing was put forward earlier than qi and yin-yang. The concept wu xing in classical Chinese philosophy evolved from the ancient concepts: "five directions" and "five materials". According to the records of oracle inscriptions of the Yin-Shang Dynasty (殷商 c. 16th-11th century B.C.) on the tortoise shells or animal bones, the Yin people (殷人) termed the Shang's territory "Center Shang", being juxtaposed to "East Land", "South Land", "West land", and "North Land". Thereby, the whole territory was divided into five parts, and then the concept of "five directions" formed.

In the late period of Western Zhou Dynasty and Spring-Autumn period (C. 1100-476 B.C.), theory of "the five directions" was followed by theory of "the five materials". Shi Bo (史伯) of the late period of Western Zhou Dynasty said that "the metal, wood, water, fire and soil are mixed to generate one hundred items" (Guo Yu •Zhen Yu, 《国语·郑语》). Zi Han (子罕) of the Spring-Autumn period said that "the heaven gives birth to the five materials. People use them together. Either can not be disposed with" (Zuo Zhuan, 《左传·襄公二十七年》).

The writing record of generalisation of the concrete material concept "five materials" to the philosophical concept "wu xing" starts with Shang Shu• Hong Fan (《尚书•洪范》), which states that "Wu xing: the first is water, the second is fire, the third is wood, the fourth is metal, the fifth is soil. Water is moistening and downward flowing. Fire is flaming upward. Wood is bending and straightening. Metal is transforming and changing. Soil, then, is sowing and reaping. Moistening and downward flowing generates salty [flavor]. Flaming upward generates bitter [flavor]. Bending and straightening generates sour [flavor]. Transforming and changing generates acrid [flavor]. Sowing and reaping generates sweet [flavor]".

In the late Warring States Period, Lu Buwei(吕不韦), the prime minister of the Qin Kingdom, compiled Lu's Spring and Autumn Annals, (Lu Shi Chun Qiu, 《吕氏春秋》), which continued to use the thinking way of Hong Fan (《洪范》), affirmed that many things in the world can be attributed to wu xing according to their qualities, and related the system of wu xing to flavors, sounds, colors, seasons, directions, internal organs, insects and domestic animals, and grains, universalised the attributes of wu xing. So, the concept of wu xing in philosophical sense had formed.

Pang Pu (庞朴) pointed out that "almost all of the thinkers of the Pre-Qin Days talked about wu xing from the record of the five directions on oracle inscriptions of the Shang Dynasty (c. 16th-11th century B.C.) on the tortoise shells or animal bones to Lu's Spring and Autumn Annals • Twelve Period (Lu Shi Chun Qiu • Shi'Er Ji) where a huge system of wu xing was established. The only difference lies in weight or significance and special aspects of wu xing in their writings" (see Pang Pu 1982, p.219).

As regard to Zou Yan (驺衍, about 305-240 B.C.), a philosopher of the late Warring States Period, Joseph Needham said, Zou Yan might not be the founder of wu xing theory, but, undoubtedly, it was he that systematised and stabilized the thinking system that had been spread for over a century (see Needham 2001, p.149).

The concept of wu xing had been used in medicine as early as the Spring-Autumn and Warring States Period to explain the attributes of internal organs and relationship among them. That is to say, introduction of the wu xing theory of philosophy to TCM is undoubtedly earlier than Huang Di's Inner Classic. A quite systematic wu xing theory has already formed in the Plain Questions (Su Wen), and all of the fives in the book evolved from wu xing, such as the five zang organs, five flavors, five colors, five qi, five essences, five spirits, five diseases, five excesses, five deficiencies, five methods, five grains, and so and so forth. For details, you may refer to the following chapters: The True Words from the Golden Chamber (Jin Kui Zhen Yan Lun, 金匮真言论), Manifestations of Yin and Yang (Yin-Yang Ying Xiang Da Lun, 阴阳应象大论), The Visceral Qi Follows the Way of the Seasons (Zang Qi Fa Shi Lun, 藏气法时论), Progression of the Wu Xing (Wu Yun Xing Da Lun, 五运行大论), etc. For example, The True Words from the Golden Chamber states that "The east and the green color correspond to the liver. The liver opens into the eyes, and the essence is stored in the liver. Illness may manifest on the head. The flavor is sour, the plant is tree/wood, the animal is the chicken, the grain is wheat, the planet is Sui/Jupiter, the number is eight, the smell is foul, the season is spring, which all pertains to the wood in wu xing. And the area affected is the tendons".[1]

3.2 Translation of "Wu Xing" in TCM

The wu xing theory, originating in China, is unique. The formation of the theory is related to the vast land of China with clear and definite five directions, clear division of the four seasons due to China's location on the North Temperate Zone, as well as rising and flourishing of the agriculture and metallurgy in the Yin-Shang Period (殷商 c. 16th-11th century B.C.) and continual stable development afterwards. Therefore, the wu xing theory thrives and does not decline.

But, "wu xing" has been mistranslated into the five elements for a long time, which is very possibly influenced by the Greek System of the

---

1   The translation accords with the interpretation and commentaries by Guo Aichun 1999, p.26

Four Elements. That is to say, translator adopts "domestication" strategy in order to make the translation more acceptable to the Western readers. Kaptchuk said that "The Five Phases are not in any way ultimate constituents of matter. This misconception has long been embodied in the common mistranslation 'Five Elements' and exemplifies the problems that arise from looking at things Chinese with a Western frame of reference. The Chinese term that we translate as 'Five Phases' is wu xing. Wu is the number five, and xing means 'walk' or 'move', and, perhaps most pertinently, it implies a process. The wu xing, therefore, are five kinds of processes; hence the Five Phases, and not the Five Elements. The theory of Phases is a system of correspondences and patterns that subsume events and things, especially in relationship to their dynamics" (see Kaptchuk 2000, p.437).

With regard to translation of wu xing, Unschuld said that "Given the development of notions of cyclical recurrences or phases of activity of the five xing, a reading of "five phases" has become popular in Western literature. In our translation we follow Harper who in his translation and discussion of the Mawangdui manuscripts adopted Marc Kalinowski's suggestion to translate wu xing as "five agents". The word agent maintains, as Harper points out, some of the material aspects of the xing as they are used in accounts of natural processes. A good medical example is the account of gestation in the Mawangdui medical text Tai chan shu (《胎产书》) where the bestowal of Water, Fire, Metal, Wood, and Earth/Soil on the fetus in the fourth through eight months of gestation enables blood, qi, muscles, bones, and skin to form" (see Unschuld 2003, p.84).

We have known that wu xing originates from the five materials, but are not the five materials whatsoever. The textbook of The Basic Theories of Chinese Medicine (5th ed. 《中医基础理论》) states that "Wu xing refers to the movement of the wood, fire, soil, metal, and water". As regard to the content of the wu xing theory, it does not discuss the specific properties of the five materials in isolation, but "has by further extension come to mean that everything in the universe comes into being by movement, change, and transformation of the five essential materials, i.e. wood, fire, soil, metal, and water", and "that engendering and restraining among wu xing are used to expound the relationship among things" (see Yin Huihe 1984, p.18).

In view of the above-mentioned facts, I suggest that wu xing be translated into five phases, five agents, or five elemental phases for "five phases" is the most popular translation for wu xing in the West, and "five agents" and "five elemental phases" maintain some of the material aspects of wu xing and can reflect the evolution process of the term wu xing to a certain extent. Moreover, the translation "five elemental phases" for wu xing is more comprehensible to the lay mind (see Lan Fengli 2003, pp.627-28).

The Greek System of the Four Elements was put forward by Empedocles (504-433 B.C., or 490-430 B.C.), a philosopher of ancient Greece. He believed that the four elements, fire, water, soil, and air, were the basic constituents of things and objects, he related the four elements to four categories like four basic properties, four humors, etc., and he also advocated that the continual change among the four elements was unceasing.[1] The following figure (see next page) shows the Greek System of the Four Elements (see Kaptchuk 2000, p.437).

Later on, Hippocratic Corpus applied the Greek System of the Four Elements to medicine, which became the system of the four humors. Hippocratic Corpus correspond the four humors to the four elements (soil, air, fire, and water), the four seasons, the four specific properties (hot, cold, damp, and dry), the four stages of human age, the four dispositions, which was used to explain the human body and pathogenesis of some diseases (see Porter 2000, p.90).

As regard to concrete medical theory, the five-agent theory in the Plain Questions and the four-humor system in the Hippocratic Corpus share some similar views. But the attributes of five agents in the Plain Questions are much wider in range than that of the four-humor system in the Hippocratic Corpus; and combined with qi and yin-yang theory, with the backing or support of visceral manifestation and meridian theories, the five-agent theory run through every link from physiology, pathology of the human being to diagnosis and treatment of diseases, thus forming a broad, circular, self-contained, integrated, and systematic theoretical system of TCM. While the four-humor system in the Hippocratic Corpus is too inferior to bear comparison.

---

1   Teaching and Research Section of History of Foreign Philosophy, Department of Philosophy, Peking University 1957, pp.73-91

blood
sanguine
heart
spring
(hot-moist)

moist   fire   hot

phlegm   yellow bile
phlegmatic   choleric
brain   water   air   liver
winter   summer
(cold-moist)   (hot-dry)

cold   earth   dry

black bile
melancholy
spleen
autumn
(cold-dry)

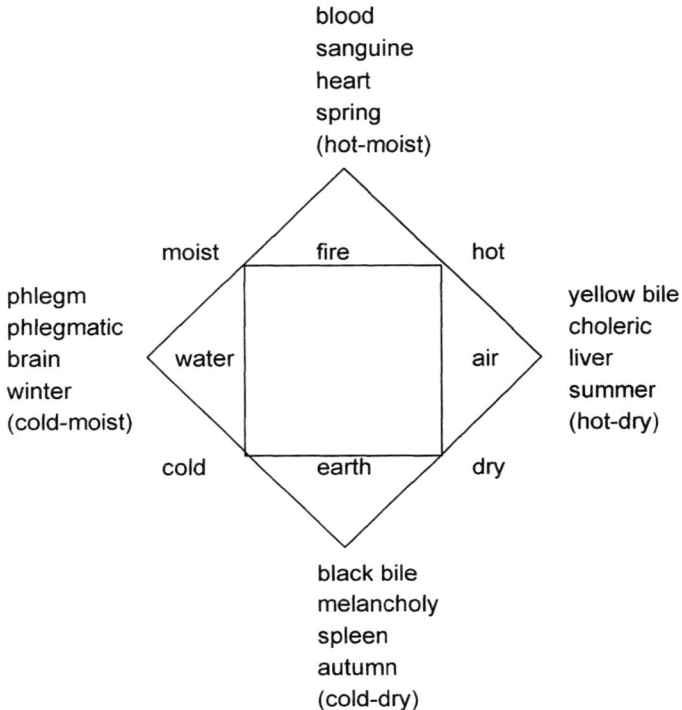

As regard to concrete medical theory, the five-agent theory in the Plain Questions and the four-humor system in the Hippocratic Corpus share some similar views. But the attributes of five agents in the Plain Questions are much wider in range than that of the four-humor system in the Hippocratic Corpus; and combined with qi and yin-yang theory, with the backing or support of visceral manifestation and meridian theories, the five-agent theory run through every link from physiology, pathology of the human being to diagnosis and treatment of diseases, thus forming a broad, circular, self-contained, integrated, and systematic theoretical system of TCM. While the four-humor system in the Hippocratic Corpus is too inferior to bear comparison.

Qi, Yin-Yang, and Five Agents are vital component parts of the theoretical system of TCM, embodying the unique thinking model of TCM.

Notes:

(1) Huang Di's Inner Classic, Huang Di Nei Jing (《黄帝内经》), comprising Plain Questions, Su Wen (《素问》), and Miraculous Pivot, Ling Shu (《灵枢》), is the earliest systematic TCM classic extant in China and has laid the foundation for the theoretical system of TCM.

(2) The medical books unearthed in the Mawangdui Han Tomb in December, 1973, Changsha, Hunan Province, include 11 books copied on silk and four books written on bamboo slips. The burying time of the tomb is 168 B.C. The books were copied about c. 3 B.C., and were the oldest TCM books in China. Most of the books are stray fragments of text without title. The books are entitled according to their contents: Prescriptions for 52 Diseases, Classic of Moxibustion with 11 Meridians of Hand and Foot, Classic of Moxibustion with 11 Yin-Yang Meridians, Methods of Pulse-Taking, Manifestations of Yin-Yang Pulse Indicating Death (The above five books comprise one volume of silk book); Que Gu Shi Qi (《却谷食气》), Classic of Moxibustion with 11 Yin-Yang Meridians (B ed.), Pictures of Taoist Breathing Exercises (The above three books comprise one volume of silk book); Methods for Preserving Health, Miscellaneous Therapies, Books on Obstetrics (The above three books comprise one volume of silk book); Ten Questions (bamboo slips), Methods of Integrating Yin and Yang (bamboo slips), Miscellaneous Contraindications (wood slips), and Supreme Way of the Land under Heaven (bamboo slips). The first five books and related achievements in research were entitled Prescriptions for 52 Diseases and published by Cultural Relics Publishing House in 1972.

(3) Treatise on Causes and Symptoms of Diseases, Zhu Bing Yuan Hou Lun (《诸病源候论》), written by Chao Yuanfang in 610 A.D., is the earliest monograph on causes and symptoms of diseases in China. It summarises medical achievements before 610, and has substantial content, including diseases of internal medicine, external medicine, gynecology, pediatrics, ENT, mouth and teeth, orthopedics and traumatology, and some infectious diseases, parasitic diseases, and surgery. It has exerted great influence on TCM of later generations.

(4) Shennong's Classic of Materia Medica, Shen Nong Ben Cao Jing(《神农本草经》), is important ancient literature on materia meidca of China, and is regarded as one of "The Four Great Classics" of TCM. The authorship was attributed to Shennong by people of the Qin-Han Era

(221B.C.-220 A.D.). The original ancient work has been lost. Its content has been preserved through quotations in the books on materia medica of the past ages. It records properties, flavors, actions and indications of 365 medicinals in detail. The thesis refers to a collection of the quotations compiled by Gu Guanguang of the Qing Dynasty.

(5) The Classic of Difficult Issues, Nanjing (《难经》), was said to be written by QinYueren (Bian Que), a famous doctor of the Warring States Period. It explains doubts on pulse-taking, meridians, zang fu organs or bowels and viscera, diseases, acupuncture points, needling techniques existing in Huang'di's Inner Classic in the form of questions and answers. It is a very important literature to study TCM.

(6) Treatise on Cold Damage, Shanghanlun (《伤寒论》), one part of Treatise on Cold Damage and Miscellaneous Diseases, Shang Han Za Bing Lun (《伤寒杂病论》), by Zhang Zhongjing of the late Eastern Han Dynasty, is the earliest and systematic literature on externally contracted febrile diseases in China, and has been playing a vital role in the development of TCM of the later generations. It has made a great advance in TCM on the basis of the theories of Nei Jing and Nan Jing by collecting effective prescriptions from all sides, incorporating the author's own clinical experiences into the book, and summarising achievements in TCM before Han Dynasty.

(7) Cambridge Illustrated History of Medicine states that the four-humor system was regarded to be founded by Hippocrates, and soon afterwards, was extended to include the four elements, i.e. soil, air, fire, and water; ... But, out of consideration for time and rationality, the four-humor system formed under the influence of the ancient Greek system of the four elements.

References

Addison Wesley Longman Limited 1998, *Longman Dictionary of Contemporary English* [Z], Beijing: The Commercial Press.
Collected by Gu Guanguang [Qing Dynasty], Textual Criticized and Annotated by Yang Pengju 2002, *ShenNong's Classic of Materia Medica*[M], Beijing: Academy Press.
Gou Aichun 1999, *Textual Criticism, Annotation and Modern Interpretation of Huang Di Nei Jing Su Wen*[M],TIanjing: Tianjin Science and Technology Press.

Kaptchuk, Ted J 2000, *Chinese Medicine: The Web That Has No Weaver* [M], Revised ed., London: Rider.

Lan Fengli 2003, Use the Translating Experiences of Other Countries for Reference to Bring about An Advance in Translation of TCM in China[J], *Chinese Journal of Integrated Traditional and Western Medicine*, 23（8）：627-28.

Lan Fengli 2005, *Cultural Connotations and English Translation of Chinese Medical Classics* (PhD Dissertation), Shanghai University of Traditional Chinese Medicine.

Lan Fengli 2006, The Influence of Huang Di's Inner Classic on The Origin of Chinese Characters[J], *Chinese Journal of Medical History*, 36(4): 201-05.

Li Jingwei, Qu Yongxin, Yu Ying'ao, et al. 2001, *A Concise Dictionary of Chinese Medicine*, Beijing: China Press of Traditional Chinese Medicine.

Li Peisheng, Cheng Zhaoren 2006, *Teaching Reference for Higher TCM Education · Shang Han Lun*[M], Beijing: People's Medica Publishing House.

Pang Pu 1982, *A Corpus of Meditation*, Shanghai: Shanghai People's Publishing House.

Teaching and Research Section of History of Foreign Philosophy, Department of Philosophy, Peking University 1957,*Philosophy of Ancient Greece and Rome*, Beijing: SDX Joint Publishing Company.

Translator: Department of History of Sciences of Shanghai Jiaotong University; Author: Needham, Joseph 2001, *Science and Civilisation in China Series* [M], Shanghai: Shanghai People's Publishing House.

Translator: Zhang Daqing; Author: Porter, Roy 2000, *The Cambridge Illustrated History of Medicine* [M], Changchun: Jilin People's Publishing House.

Unschuld, Paul U 2003, *HUANG DI NEI JING SU WEN: Nature, Knowledge, Imagery in An Ancient Chinese Medical Text* [M], Berkeley, Los Angeles and London: University of California Press.

Veith, Ilza 1949, *The Yellow Emperor's Classic of Internal Medicine*. 1st Ed., Baltimore: The Williams & Wilkins Co.

Veith, Ilza 1966, 1972, *The Yellow Emperor's Classic of Internal Medicine*. 2nd ed., Berkeley, Los Angeles, London: University of California Press.

Webster's Encyclopedic Unabridged Dictionary of the English Language (New Revised Edition) [Z], New York: Gramercy Books, 1994.

Xie Zhufan 2002, *Classified Dictionary of Traditional Chinese Medicine* [Z], Beijing: Foreign Languages Press.

Yin Huihe 1984, *Textbook for TCM Higher Education · The Basic Theories of Traditional Chinese Medicine*, Shanghai: Shanghai Scientific and Technological Publisher.

Wang Xin-Yuan & Pu Gong-Ying

Lemology in Traditional Chinese Medicine: With Prevention and Treatment of SARS as A Case in Point

Translated by Lan Fengli

In the spring of 2003, SARS (Severe Acute Respiratory Syndrome) suddenly broke out and affected the whole world. After making a general survey of the history, we know that acute infectious diseases accompany the development of civilisation of human beings. Serious prevalence may even last for about one hundred years, change the progress of history, exterminate an ethnic group, or destroy a country, thus resulting in extremely big damage. And how does the traditional Chinese medicine deal with them?

1. History and Reality

As early as in Zhou Dynasty (C.1100-256 B.C.) in China, record on infectious disease began to appear. According to the statistics of *A Chronology of Chinese Medical History* (《中国医史年表》), over 300 big spreads of infectious diseases were recorded up till 1949. Among them, outbreaks of infectious diseases were most in the Qing Dynasty (1644-1911), accounting for 2/5. As regards to the law of the attack of infectious diseases, Chinese ancestors summarised that "a big war or disaster must be followed by a serious epidemic". Taking a sweeping view of the history, records on infectious diseases are indeed present more in turbulent dynasties such as Eastern Han (25-220A.D.), Three Kingdoms (220-265A.D.), Southern Song (1127-1279), Ming (1368-1644) and Qing (1644-1911) Dynasties. For instance, Zhang Zhong-Jing (张仲景) stated in the preface of the *Treatise on Cold-Induced and Miscellaneous Diseases* (《伤寒杂病论·序》) that 2/3 of his patriarchal clan with over 200 members died of successive years of epidemic diseases.

Traditional Chinese medicine has been the pillar to fight against infectious diseases in China for thousands of years. In TCM, virulent infectious disease is also known as pestilence, seasonal contagious disease, etc. In the *Plain Questions ·Needling Techniques* (《素问遗篇刺法论》), it is stated that "the attack of five types of infectious diseases spreads to all the people, no matter young or old, with similar symptoms". As regards to the forecast, prevention, diagnosis, treatment of infectious diseases, TCM is complete in theory, abundant in therapeutic methods, and the therapeutic effects are generally acknowledged by the common people. Prominent physicians on epidemiology have been coming forth in large numbers in the history, such as Zhang Zhong-Jing, the sage in TCM, of the Eastern Han Dynasty, Sun Si-Miao (孙思邈), the king of medicine, of the Tang Dynasty (618-907), Wu You-Ke (吴又可) of the Ming Dynasty, Yu Shi-Yu (余师愚) and Wang Meng-Ying (王孟英) of the Qing Dynasty, Kong Bo-Hua (孔伯华) and Pu Fu-Zhou (蒲辅周) of the modern times, and so and so forth. The works reflecting the achievements on epidemiology are as follows: the classical works such as *The Inner Classic* (nei jing, 《内经》), *Treatise on Cold-Induced Diseases* (shang han lun, 《伤寒论》); works on prescriptions such as *A Handbook of Prescriptions for Emergencies* (zhou hou jiu cu fang, 《肘后救卒方》), *Invaluable Prescriptions* (qian jin fang, 《千金方》), *Medical Secrets of An Official* (wai tai mi yao, 《外台秘要》), *Prescriptions for Universal Relief* (pu ji fang, 《普济方》), *Liu He-Jian's Six books of Medicine* (he jian liu shu, 《河间六书》), *The Confucians' Care of Their Parents* (ru men shi qin, 《儒门事亲》), *Compendium of Chinese Materia Medica* (ben cao gang mu, 《本草纲目》), *An Outline of Epidemic Febrile Diseases* (wen re jing wei, 《温热经纬》), etc.; monographs on lemology such as *Treatise on Pestilences* (wen yi lun, 《瘟疫论》), *Analysis of Cold-Induced Diseases and Pestilences* (shan han wen yi tiao bian, 《伤寒瘟疫条辨》), etc. The following are some successful cases of dealing with infectious diseases in the history of TCM.

In the April of 1202, many people suffered from an infectious disease, first, manifesting in such symptoms as aversion to cold, or fever, or body heaviness without fever, then in severe swollen head and face, eyes being unable to open, panting, sore throat, dry mouth and tongue, which was diagnosed as "swollen-head infection" (erysipelas facialis) in TCM. There was a saying that most of the patients with "swollen-head infection" would die of it. Li Dong-Yuan (李东垣), one of the four great physicians in the Jin-Yuan Dynasties (1115-1368), believed that the disease is caused by pathogenic heat invading the space between the heart and lungs, then attacking the head and face, thus causing severe swollen head. He then formulated a formula named Universal Antitoxic Decoction (pu ji xiao du yin zi, 普济消毒饮子), which cured many patients of the disease and was regarded as a "fairy formula".

In Qianlong's reign of the Qing Dynasty, severe pestilence broke out in Beijing. Yu Shi-Yu (余师愚), a famous physician from Tong-Cheng city, cured numerous patients by administering a prescription containing a large dosage of gypsum. [*An Outline of Epidemic Febrile Diseases* (wen re jing wei, 《温热经纬》)]

In 1956, encephalitis B was prevalent in Shijiazhuang, Hebei province. Zhang Zhong-Jing's White Tiger Decoction (bai hu tang, 白虎汤) was administered to patients, and the achieved therapeutic effects surpassed the world levels although no theories on microorganisms ever exist in TCM. In 1957, encephalitis B was prevalent in Beijing. But the White Tiger Decoction did not yield notable effects. Pu Fu-Zhou (蒲辅周), a prominent physician in Beijing, added Rhizoma Atractylodis (cang zhu, 苍术) to eliminate dampness according to the theory of five circuit phases and six climatic factors and the humid climate of that year, which achieved 90 per cent rate of efficiency. In 1968, encephalitis B was prevalent in Guangzhou, Guangdong province. Deng Tie-Tao (邓铁涛), a prominent physician, identified the disease as the pattern of summer heat with latent dampness, and gave patients corresponding prescriptions. Statistics showed that the rate of efficiency of TCM reached 90 per cent, and moreover, TCM therapies did not yield any side-effect.

In 2003, Guangdong Hospital of TCM achieved amazing therapeutic effects in preventing and treating SARS according to the TCM theory of Spring Warm, i.e. febrile disease in the spring. It was reported in the Guang-Ming Daily (guang ming ri bao, April 29th) that the experiences in preventing and treating SARS of Guangdong province demonstrated that TCM is remarkably effective in preventing and treating the disease. The No. 1 Hospital Affiliated to Guangzhou University of TCM adopted TCM therapies to treat SARS after physicians of Western medicine made a definite diagnosis of SARS for altogether 36 cases, and achieved markedly therapeutic effect. Up till April 14th, no patient died, most of the patients were discharged from hospital after recovery without any aftereffect; the average time of allaying fever was three days, and the average time of hospitalisation was no more than nine days; no medical care worker was affected. Experts of World Health Organisation (WHO) highly appraised the satisfactory therapeutic effects of TCM in treating SARS and suggested to improve such clinical experiences to a level of routine treatment, thus helping other countries prevent and treat it. TCM experts from the first-line work of fighting SARS of Guangdong province pointed out that TCM can eliminate such pathogenic factors as dampness and heat toxin, arousing capability of self-organisation of the human beings, fighting disease and "killing enemies", thus curing SARS, through the way of pattern identification and treatment. TCM has its specific strong points in dealing with disease whose pathogen is still unclear. It is also worth to note that early application of TCM prescriptions can block the further progressing of the disease.

Both the history and reality have proved that TCM have successfully resolved prevention and treatment of various infectious diseases and made great contributions to the living and multiplying of the Chinese people.

2. Theory on Lemology

TCM holds that pestilence results from interaction of multiple factors involving the human being itself, and the outside environment of the heaven and earth, i.e., the nature. *The Inner Classic* clarifies the influence of the five circuit phases and six climatic factors on the human being. (See the two chapters of the *Plain Question* missing and subsequently added to it (su wen yi pian, 《素问遗篇》) for details on interaction of the heaven, earth and human being in the occurrence of infectious diseases.) TCM can grasp various factors in the occurrence of infectious diseases, and then seize the general law of infectious diseases and the characteristics of each attack.

2.1 Etiology

TCM holds that the cause of pestilence is the turbid qi in between the heaven and earth. Wu You-Ke's *Treatise on Pestilences* states that "the cause of pestilence is not wind, cold, summer-heat, or dampness, but an unusual qi or pestilential qi in between the heaven and earth". But Wu did not intend to seek cause or therapeutic method outside the system of TCM. In the *Yan Jing Yan* (《研经言》) it is stated that "there are altogether six kinds of qi or six climatic factors in between the heaven and earth, the thick factors are pestilential qi which are toxic. Toxin refers to the thick characteristics of qi". Of course, pestilence is not simply caused by the six climatic pathogenic factors, but its etiology cannot be separated from them.

In the *Magical Effects of Contemporary Formulas* (shi fang miao yong 《时方妙用》), it is stated that "the etiology of seasonal epidemics may be of two ways. One is from the heaven, i.e. climatic pathogenic factors. For instance, the spring should be warm but cold instead, the summer should be hot but cool instead, the autumn should be cool but hot instead, and the winter should be cold but warm instead, which is called "the climate presents in improper season". Such climatic pathogenic factors attack the human beings through meridians or channels, causing headache, fever, cough, or swollen neck, or suppurative parotitis, or swollen-head wind, etc., which are the infectious diseases caused by the climatic pathogenic factors. The other is the pestilential qi from the patient and has nothing to do with the heaven or climatic pathogenic factors. It is like this. One patient's disease spreads to his/her roommates or family members, then to the village, then to the entire town. The pestilential qi infects others through the nose and mouth, and manifests itself in such symptoms as aversion to cold, high fever, fullness and oppression in the chest and diaphragm, expectoration of yellowish saliva.

2.2 Law of Transmission and Change of Pestilence

Chen Xiu-Yuan (陈修园) said that "there are two ways for pestilence to enter the body, i.e. the meridians and the nose and mouth, but the transmission and change of the pestilence follow the same six-meridian law as that of the cold-induced disease or externally contracted febrile disease". In the *Extensive Treatise on Pestilence* (guang wen yi lun, 《广瘟疫论》) it is stated that "transmission of pestilence through meridians is different from that of wind-cold. The wind-cold transmits from the exterior to the interior, so it must spread from Great Yang (taiyang) to Yang Brightness (yangming), then to Lesser Yang (shaoyang), and then enter the stomach in the interior; while pestilence starts from the middle way by exiting the exterior and entering the interior, transmits and changes according to the weak or the strong of the qi in different meridians. Therefore, Wu You-Ke said that pestilential pathogen may transmit from the exterior to the interior, or from the interior to the exterior, may manifest itself only in the exterior, or only in the interior, may manifest itself in more exterior pattern, or in more interior pattern, may manifest itself in exterior pattern again and again, or in interior pattern again and again, may transmit to the exterior and interior respectively, which are altogether known as nine transmissions". Pattern identification according to the six-meridian, wei-defense, qi, ying-construction, and blood, as well as the triple burner, the different level systems of the human being can all be used to treat infectious diseases.

2.3 Treatment of Pestilence

In the *Triple-Character Bible for Medicine* (yi xue sanzi jing, 《医学三字经》) it is stated that "Ginseng Toxin-Removing Powder (ren shen bai du san , 人参败毒散) can be used to treat the infectious disease in its initial stage accompanied by the symptom of aversion to cold where pathogen enters the body through meridian to support healthy qi and dispel pathogenic factors, and that Health-restoring Agastache Powder (huo xiang zheng qi san , 藿香正气散) can be used to treat the infectious disease in its initial stage accompanied by the symptom of chest fullness, expectoration of yellowish saliva where pathogen attacks the body through the nose and mouth to resolve bad pathogen by the use of acrid aromatics, and that Miraculous Powder of Saposhnikovia (fang feng tong sheng san , 防风通圣散) can provide full treatment for the disease without the side effect of inducing pathogen towards the interior".

In the *Magical Effects of Contemporary Formulas* (shi fang miao yong 《时方妙用》) it is stated that "among the infectious diseases caused by invasion of climatic pathogenic factors into the body through meridians, the disease of the cold pattern should be treated with Five-Accumulation

Powder (Wu Ji San, 五积散) of acrid and warm in nature; The disease of heat pattern should be given Nine-Ingredient Decoction with Notopterygium (jiu wei qiang huo tang, 九味羌活汤). If qi is in deficiency, sweating can not be used, and Ginseng Toxin-Removing Powder (ren sheng bai du san) should be given to treat the disease. High fever resists pathogens, sweating can not be induced and Miraculous Powder of Saposhnikovia (fang feng tong sheng san) is appropriate. Suppurative parotitis and swollen head syndrome caused by toxin of wind-fire should be treated with Miraculous Powder of Saposhnikovia (fang feng tong sheng san) plus Fructus Viticis (niu bang zi, 牛蒡子), Flos Lonicerae (jin yin hua, 金银花), Radix Platycodi (jie geng, 桔梗), Bulbus Fritillarie Ussuriensis (bei mu, 贝母), and Fructus Trichosanthis (gua lou ren, 瓜蒌仁). The pathogenic factors should be induced out through meridians with the method of sweating for they enter the body through meridians.

"Among the infectious diseases caused by invasion of pestilential qi from patient into the body through the nose and mouth, Cyperus and Perilla Drink (xiang su yin, 香苏饮) plus Rhizoma Polygonati Odorati (yu zhu, 玉竹), Rhizoma Chuanxiong (chuan xiong, 川芎), and Caulis Lonicerae (ren dong, 忍冬), or Wondrous Atractylodes Powder (shen zhu san, 神术散) plus Radix Puerariae (ge gen, 葛根) and Onion (cong tou, 葱头), or Health-restoring Agastache Powder (huo xiang zheng qi san, 藿香正气散) can be used to treat this type of diseases. The pathogenic factors should be induced out through the nose and mouth for they enter the body through them."

"If the pathogenic agent is transmitted to the Yang Brightness (yangming) meridians from meridians or from the nose and mouth and manifests itself in such symptoms as spontaneous sweating, great thirsty and profuse sweating, Sweet Dew Beverage (gan lu yin, 甘露饮) should be used to engender liquid so as to defeat pathogenic agent and bring the patient back to life; if the condition is severe, Ginseng White Tiger Decoction (bai hu ren sheng tang, 白虎人参汤) must be used to clear the scattered heat in the Yang Brightness (yangming) meridians so as to induce heat out of the body."

"If the pathogenic agent enters the stomach, delirious speech, mania, dry stool, and the lower abdomen refusing pressure will be present, and Three-in-One Qi-Coordinating Decoction (san yi cheng qi tang, 三一承气

汤) is appropriate. When there is excess heat in the interior and excess pathogenic agent in the exterior, Miraculous Powder of Saposhnikovia (fang feng tong sheng san), the most effective formula in treating infectious disease, should be used to resolve them together."

"If people of weak constitution suffers from infectious disease, or prolonged disease or malpractice makes patient in debility, the modified Four Agents Decoction (si wu tang，四物汤), Four Gentlemen Decoction (si jun zi tang，四君子汤), Center-Supplementing Qi-Boosting Decoction (bu zhong yi qi tang，补中益气汤) should be used to supplement, nourish the healthy qi so as to express the pathogenic agent."

"In a word, infectious diseases must be resolved through great sweating. A patient of a strong physique will perspire without shivering. A patient of a weak physique must shiver first and perspire afterwards. ... The key to treat infectious disease is to cause sweating. If sweating is induced, the patient will be cured of the disease; if sweating can not be induced, the patient will die. Malpractice such as the treatment which dries up the source of sweat or forces to sweat will make patient die unclear of the false practice."

In the *Therapeutic Methods for Damp-Warm and Seasonal Epidemic* (shi wen shi yi zhi liao fa，《湿温时疫治疗法》. Damp-warm refers to an infectious febrile disease caused by damp-heat.) It records some methods to deal with infectious diseases:

First, keep the clothes and quilts clean. Sanitation and hygiene are essential for all the diseases, esp. for infectious diseases. Otherwise, infectious diseases will spread to the patient's family and physician(s) as well. Therefore, the patient should change his/her clothes everyday, and the bedding must be maintained clean. If the patient is covered too many quilts, he/she will be too hot, his/her condition will be aggravated, and death may even ensue for the heat stagnates inside and qi fails to disperse.

Second, be moderate in eating and drinking. Damp-warm and seasonal epidemic are originally caused by latent pathogen in the stomach and intestines. The patient has already suffered from indigestion, can endure hunger, and should lie on the bed and keep quiet. Greasy, sea, roast, raw and cold food, as well as melons and fruits should not be taken in. The soup made of radish and dried vegetable is best for it can remove obstructions in the stomach and intestines. When the patient becomes better, he can take in some fluid nourishing food, such as thin gruel made of rice or lotus root paste, or egg custard. The patient should take less food in one meal and have more meals a day. All foods which are difficult to be digested such as unripe fruits, oily and solid foods should not be taken in before the patient has fully recovered from the disease. Pang An-chang (庞安常) said that when the patient has just recovered from the disease, he/she should be given only thin rice gruel, then thick rice gruel afterwards and both in a quite small amount, and should not be given meat, wine, sweet, greasy, uncooked and cold food. Wang Meng-ying (王孟英) said that when the sufferer recovers from the disease, his/her urine and tongue coating will be both clear, then the patient can be allowed to take some gruel; Wine, sweet, greasy and fresh food can be given step by step only after dry and new stool is discharged from the body; otherwise, other disease may ensue. Both quotations are famous and effective ways of eating gained from their own experiences for the care of the patient.

Third, select a big room as the patient's bedroom, and open the windows to ventilate the room. Keeping the air inside the room being fresh is of prime importance in sanitation.

Fourth, it's not necessary to arrange too many people to look after the patient. If there were too many people in the patient's bedroom, the air inside the room should be easy to get stale, the patient's condition would certainly aggravate, or even die of the disease.

Fifth, make sure the doctor you select has sound credentials, and trust him/her from beginning to end. Wang Meng-ying said that to select a qualified doctor is more difficult than to select a good general; some doctor may just have a false reputation and no real learning, or may be learned but not versatile, or may be an all-rounded person without judicious judgment, or may have keen insight and no courage and resourcefulness, or may have courage ad no careful consideration to patient; all of the above-mentioned doctors can not cure serious diseases; So how dare to follow and take their prescriptions? If a doctor inquires the patient very comprehensively, gives the patient very careful consideration, identifies the patient's pattern accurately, determines treatment and prescription very clearly, his wording is straightforward and reasonable, his behavior is natural and at ease, he will be a good doctor at first sight, so his prescription can be followed and taken. Zhou Xue-qiao (周雪樵) said that the honor or disgrace of the doctor relies on the safety and well-being of the patient; If the patient can trust a doctor from the beginning to end, the doctor and the patient will have an intimate relationship between each other; if the patient seeks medical help from different doctors for the same disease even in just one day, each doctor sticks to his own point of view and administers his own different treatment and prescription, the mixture of administration of cool and warm treatments will not exert any therapeutic effect and you do not know which doctor should be blamed for; the most indignant is that the patient who only knows a little medicine is the largest resistance to a good doctor in curing the disease for he dare not take potent or strong prescriptions so as not to be maltreated and he will take mild prescription at ease and put the blame on the doctor if it is not effective. Therefore, good doctors will not be tainted with patients' bad habits but enlighten them instead.

Sixth, be cautious about inspecting and buying Chinese medicinal substances to avoid false ones. Xu Hui-xi (徐洄溪) said that a doctor should provide medicinal substances for patients and not buy them from the market in order to avoid false ones. The false medicinal substances will not exert any therapeutic effect even if the disease pattern is accurately identified and prescription is properly administered. For example, Mrs. Chen's son of Tongxiang county town suffered from cholera and asked a doctor to administer a prescription which contained 6g of prepared Rhizoma Pinelliae (zhi ban xia, 制半夏). Then the family went to a pharmacy to fill in the prescription. At that time, there were fewer shop assistants and many buyers in the pharmacy, the prepared Radix Aconiti Lateralis (zhi fu zi, 制附子) was dispensed instead of prepared Rhizoma Pinelliae (zhi ban xia). The patient suffered from sharp and severe abdominal pain and mania immediately after taking the decoction, then his mouth bled, finally the patient died. Mrs. Chen attributed her son's death to the doctor, and the doctor said the prescription was right and there must be some other reasons. Then he asked to inspect the residues of the decoction and found Radix Aconiti Lateralis (fu zi) instead of Rhizoma Pinelliae (ban xia) in it, then brought a suit against the pharmacy, finally the pharmacy paid some money to compensate Mrs. Chen for loss of her son and end the conflict.

3. Prevention of Pestilence

Of course, prevention of infectious diseases is the most important! In the Chapter of Regulating the Spirit in Accordance With the Four Seasons (si qi tiao shen da lun , 四气调神大论) of the *Su Wen*, or Plain Questions, it is stated that "the sages treated disease by preventing illness before it began, just as a good government or emperor was able to take the necessary steps to avert war. Treating an illness after it has begun is like suppressing revolt after it has broken out. If someone digs a well when thirsty, or forges weapons after being engaged in battle, one cannot help but ask: "Are not these actions too late?" The Chinese people, the descendants of Yan Di and Huang Di, the two legendary rulers of remote antiquity, have accumulated plentiful methods to prevent infectious diseases through thousands of years of practice, which need the modern people to carry on.

TCM believes that infectious disease is caused by bad qi, so supporting healthy qi, dispelling pathogenic factors, and removing toxin can be used to prevent infectious disease. First of all, regulating diet and life style and various methods of conducting exercise should be used to activate healthy qi of the body so as to prevent infectious disease. Then, use of fiery medicine of pure yang in nature like realgar (xiong huang，雄黄) and aromatics to refute bad qi like orchid and Radix Angelica Dahuricae (bai zhi，白芷) should be used to prevent infectious disease.

In the *Therapeutic Methods for Damp-Warm* (infectious febrile disease caused by damp-heat) *and* Seasonal *Epidemic*（shi wen shi yi zhi liao fa）, it is stated that in the prevalence of seasonal epidemic, people should have a regular life style, balanced diet, and be moderate on sexual activities.

The methods of preventing infectious disease recorded in ancient TCM texts can be summarised as follows:

3.1 Method of Inspecting, Meditating, and Conducting Exercise

The chapter of Needing Techniques（ci fa lun, 刺法论）of *Huang Di Nei Jing Su Wen* recorded the method of inspecting and meditating the five *zang* organs emitting five colors to protect the body by maintaining healthy qi inside and preventing epidemic from entering the body.

3.2 Medication

In the chapter of Needing Techniques （ci fa lun） of *Huang Di Nei Jing Su Wen* it is stated that at the day of the Spring Equinox, two cups of decoction of Radix Polygalae (yuan zhi，远志) with the core removed should be taken when facing the east to induce vomiting to prevent the occurrence of epidemic disease.

In the *Invaluable Prescriptions for Emergencies* (bei ji qian jin yao fang, 《备急千金要方》) it is stated that Fructus Cannabis (ma zi ren, 麻子仁) and Semen Phaseoli (chi xiao dou，赤小豆) should be taken 14 grains respectively in the morning to prevent infectious disease.

3.3 External Application

In the chapter of Needling Techniques (ci fa lun) of *Huang Di Nei Jing Su Wen* it is recorded a medicinal formula for bathing to induce sweating to prevent disease. External application of Fen Shen Powder (粉身散) is recorded in the *Invaluable Prescriptions for Emergencies* (bei ji qian jin yao fang) to prevent infectious disease.

3.4 Burning and Fumigating

A Ghost-Killing Burning Prescription to avoid pestilential qi is recorded in the *Invaluable Prescriptions for Emergencies* (bei ji qian jin yao fang):
Realgar (xiong huang，雄黄) 500g   Cinnabaris (zhu sha，朱砂) 500g Orpiment (ci huang，雌黄) 500g   Cornu Saigae Tataricae （羚羊角） 150g   Semen Torreyae (wu yi 芜荑, fei zi 榧子) 150g   Tiger Bone 150g Rhizoma Dysosmac Versipellis (gui jiu，鬼臼) 150g   Herba Buchnerae (gui jian yu, 鬼箭羽) 150g   Radix Pulsatillae (bai tou weng，白头翁) 150g   adiantum (shi chang sheng，石长生) 150g   Maxuanti （马悬蹄）150g   Goat fat （qing yang zhi, 青羊脂）240g   Rhizoma Acori Tatarinowii (chang pu, 菖蒲) 240g Rhizoma Atractylodis Macrocephalae (bai zhu，白术) 240g Amber 4000g

Grind them into powder, make the powder into pellet size pill with the amber, then burn it in the morning and evening in front of the home.

Aromatics, such as natural white sandalwood, Chinese eagle wood, or senior joss stick, can also be burned to avoid pestilential qi in the daily life.

The history and reality have proved that various infectious diseases are not new to Chinese medicine and that Chinese medicine has already well resolved prevention and treatment of pestilence, thus making a tremendous contribution to multiplication of Chinese nationality unparallel in history. But can these economic, effective, and precious methods be applied to prevent and treat pestilence?

4. Practical Experience

In April of 2003, the author had the opportunity to diagnose and treat SARS patients directly with TCM in isolation wards and achieved a quite satisfactory result. Of 15 cases, no death was reported, the mild cases were all cured and the severe cases were all improved. Thereafter, some understanding and thoughts occurred to me.

Both "SARS" (Severe Acute Respiratory Syndrome) and "Atypical Pneumonia" are disease names in the Western medicine. From the perspective of Chinese medicine, the disease should be certainly attributed to "pestilence". After reviewing the TCM classics and the theory of five circuit phases and six climatic factors, the author found that in the chapter of Comprehensive Discourse on the Policies and Arrangements of the Six Originals or The Six Macrocosmic Influences (liu yuan zheng ji da lun, 六元正纪大论) of Huang Di Nei Jing Su Wen it is stated that "whenever the Great Yin or Taiyin controls the heaven energy and plays its role ... In the stage of the second energy or qi (March to May of the solar calendar), the monarch fire is playing its role, all things are being bred and transformed, and people are in a harmonious state. As the fire is abundant, the pestilence will be prevalent far and near". The year of 2003 is the very year when the Great Yin or Taiyin (damp –earth) controls the heaven energy and plays its role. A conclusion could be drawn through a comprehensive consideration of clinical observation, climate and geographical features: SARS was a kind of pestilence caused by dampness and heat, which was easy and quick to spread, transmit, change, block the qi dynamic, and damage the lungs.

134

Why was the northern China affected by dampness and heat? Besides the Great Yin or Taiyin (damp –earth) controlling the heaven energy and playing its role, the influence of the heaven and earth was another reason. Kong Bo-Hua (孔伯华), a noted physician in Beijing, said that "my dozens of years of experiences showed that about 80-90 per cent patients' diseases were caused by dampness and heat …", and that "why was there so much dampness-heat? Was it caused by the influence of the heaven and earth? From the perspective of the cycle of the sixty years, the sequence of the four seasons was abnormal, yang was in hyperactivity and yin was in deficiency, dampness-heat permeated and was in excess. Therefore, the acrid, warm, enriching and greasy medicinals should be used very cautiously. Yin was always in deficiency and yang was always in excess. When fire and heat were mixed, dampness would be transformed into heat".

The diseases were all caused by direct invasion of dampness-heat and turbid pathogens into the lung meridian through the nose and mouth in over thirty patients the author had experienced.

Stagnant heat is in the lung meridian and dampness obstructs the qi dynamic. If the dampness and heat do not integrate each other, the heat pathogen together with the dampness will attack the body, manifesting in fever, slight aversion to cold, sore throat, dry or sticky mouth, dry cough or oppression in the chest, or poor appetite, difficulty in defecation. The tongue is red, the coating is whitish and greasy, and the pulse is floating and soggy coating. Resolving the exterior with acrid and cool medicinals, clearing heat and transforming dampness are appropriate therapeutic methods. Lonicera and Forsythia Powder (yin qiao san, 银翘散) plus Herba Agastachis (huo xiang, 藿香) Herba Eupatorii (pei lan, 佩兰), and Rhizome Imperatae (bai mao gen, 白茅根) can be prescribed for patients.

If the dampness and heat have integrated with each other, the clinical manifestations are as follows: afternoon fever, seldom aversion to cold, heaviness and pain in the body and head, sticky mouth without thirst, dry cough, feeling of oppression in the chest, poor appetite, difficulty in defecation, loose stool, and red tongue with white, thick, and greasy coating. The pulse may be wiry, fine and soggy or deep and fine. The heat pathogen is of yang in nature and the dampness pathogen is of yin in nature. The integration of both pathogens is just like the oil entering the dough, which is sentimentally attached to each other. In the *Analysis of Warm Diseases* (wen bing tiao bian) it is stated that the disease pattern is very much like the pattern of yin deficiency, but sweating, precipitating, and moistening methods should be contraindicated in this pattern. Dispersing the upper energizer, freeing the middle energizer, and disinhibiting the lower energizer are appropriate therapeutic methods. Modified three kernels decoction (三仁汤) should be prescribed for the patients.

The above patterns are mild. Most of the patients of these patterns can be cured after taking appropriate prescriptions and will not transform into severe ones.

If the pathogenic damp-heat lingers on the qi stage, the symptoms and signs such as high fever which aggravates in the afternoon, heaviness in the body, red tongue with yellowish and greasy coating, fine, deep and rapid pulse will manifest, and modified Sweet Dew Toxin-Dispersing Elixir (gan lu xiao du dan, 甘露消毒丹) will exert a satisfactory effect. Wang Meng-Ying (王孟英), an expert in Warm Disease of the Qing Dynasty, said that "Sweet Dew Toxin-Dispersing Elixir (gan lu xiao du dan) is the chief formula to treat seasonal epidemic caused by pathogenic damp-warm. ... When the patient's tongue coating is pale white, or thick greasy, or dry yellowish, which indicates that the pathogenic summer-heat, dampness, heat, and pestilential qi are still at the qi stage, this formula will exert an immediate therapeutic effect". (*An Outline of Epidemic Febrile Diseases*, wen re jing wei)

The extremely severe cases the author saw were mostly caused by pathogenic dampness, heat, and phlegm obstructing the lungs, the lung qi being stagnated and blocked and failed to be dispersed, finally resulting in lung blockage disease, manifesting in oppression or pain in the chest, severe panting or labored breathing, dry cough, sputum being difficult to be expectorated, lassitude, lack of strength, red tongue with yellowish, thick and greasy coating, and deep, fine and rapid pulse. If these cases were not treated, they would worsen, and the prognosis would be very unfavorable. Most of the death cases were the results of the severe cases.

In the chapter of the Upper Energizer of *Analysis of Warm Diseases* (wen bing tiao bian) it is stated that "Thousand Gold Pieces Phragmites Decoction (qian jin wei jing tang, 千金苇茎汤) plus Semen Armeniacae Amarum (xing ren，杏仁) and Talcum (hua shi，滑石) can be adopted for damp-warm disease in the Great Yin (tai yin) with panting and short breath". The prescription is as follows: Rhizoma Phragmitis (lu gen，芦根) 15g, Semen Coicis (yi yi ren，薏苡仁) 15g, Semen Persicae (tao ren，桃仁) 6g, Semen Benincasa Hispida (dong gua zi，冬瓜子) 6g, Semen Armeniacae Amarum (xing ren，杏仁) 9g, Talcum (hua shi，滑石) 9g. Herba Agastachis (huo xiang，藿香), Herba Eupatorii (pei lan，佩兰), and Radix Curcumae (yu jin，郁金) can be added according to the patient's condition. Most of the severe cases will take a turn for the better and be out of danger after taking the decoction. What is the mechanism of the decoction? An Outline of Epidemic Febrile Diseases (wen re jing wei) states that, Rhizoma Phragmitis (lu gen，芦根) is similar to the pulmonary tubes in morphology, sweet in taste and cool in nature, can clear the lungs; besides, it has some joints and grows in the water, but can not be blocked by the fluids. Therefore, it can free the way in the cases where the blockage of fluids results in diseases. Semen Coicis (yi yi ren，薏苡仁), white in color, bland in taste, cool in nature, and downbearing in action, corresponds to the metal in the five elemental phases, therefore, can be used to nourish the lung qi to clear and downbear (heat and dampness). It can not be without for all the cases of invasion of pathogenic damp-heat into the lungs. Semen Benincasa Hispida (dong gua zi，冬瓜子) comes from the pulp, but can preserve its vital qi in the pulp; Therefore, it can also restore healthy qi for the patient and is good at treating mass and abscess in the abdomen to flush abscess, blood, turbidity, and phlegm. Semen Persicae (tao ren，桃仁) is said to enter the blood aspect and can free qi. So, the prescription is not only a miraculous cure for pulmonary abscess, but can also be used to cure severe pulmonary impediment (or pulmonary blockage disease).

The previously stated symptoms are just the common ones in transition and change of disease. In fact, different symptoms may occur due to various constitutions of patients and the influence of differentiated treatments. Doctor should "take the pulse and determine its type in order to know the invading pathogen and treat it according to the pattern." (Treatise on Cold-Induced Diseases, shang han lun). For instance, Mr. Li, 40 years old, had no high fever after the occurrence of disease with anorexia, nausea, stomachache and loose stool caused by the deficiency of the spleen and stomach as well as the pestilent pathogen which became coldness and lingered in the middle energizer. He was cured by modified Health-restoring Agastache Powder (huo xiang zheng qi san，藿香正气散). Mrs. Fu, 40 years old, overused cool and cold medicine which induced diarrhea seven to eight times in one day, accompanied by panting and hurried pulse. *Treatise on Cold-Induced Diseases* (shang han lun) states that "Pueraria, Scutellaria, and Coptis Decoction (gegen huangqin huanglian tang, 葛根黄芩黄连汤) is indicated in the cases with unresolved exterior pattern and hurried pulse, panting and sweating". Her symptoms were alleviated when treated accordingly.

Doctor should inspect tongue and take pulse of the patients with bloody phlegm and snivel. If the pathogen has yet transmitted to the nutrient and blood aspects, the previous formula needs to be modified by removing acrid and warm medicine which tend to stir blood and adding blood-cooling medicine. Some noticeable points:

Tonifying medicine should not be abused. Excessive dampness resembles deficient pattern in its manifestation although it's mainly excessive pattern induced by exogenous pathogen. Abusing tonifying medicine may block the pathogen inside and strengthen it. Even when the healthy qi is too weak to combat the pathogen, doctor should prescribe only a little tonifying medicine which doesn't eliminate the pathogen. Sweet and warm medicine with the tendency of blocking and sour medicine with the tendency of astringing are absolutely forbidden. Tonifying medicine can be applied when disease is about to be cured and pathogen be eliminated.

Cool and cold medicine cannot be applied without deliberation. Dampness is a pathogenic factor of yin nature, tending to stagnate qi movement. The application of cool and cold medicine which tends to astringe and stagnate may further block the qi movement, possibly impelling the invasion of pathogen. "When the pathogen is in the exterior, diaphoretics can be applied."(*Treatise on Epidemic Febrile Diseases*, Wen Re Lun) It's worth heed especially during the early stage of disease.

"The treatment of the upper energizer is as light as the feather." If the symptoms occur in the upper energizer, the nature and quantity of applied medicine should be light in order to target at the morbid location.

During the paroxysm of disease, pathogenic qi is likely to stir blood and thus the blood-activating medicine should be used cautiously.

5. Afterthoughts and Appeal

After this practice, reviewing the TCM classics and recalling the history of epidemic prevention, we find that all the previous sages of TCM strictly comply with the motto "Studying the past experience diligently and applying various prescriptions extensively" and TCM theories while incorporating distinctions of different times and consideration of time, location and person into their treatment. The flexibility of their treatments attains remarkable results.

The experience of Guangdong, the clinical practice in Beijing and personal experience of the writer prove that complying with TCM theories can bring about favorable results while defying it with a maverick's view may be failed. It also indicates from both positive and negative aspects that TCM theories reflect the objective truth and thus these theories are scientific and have to be observed.

Now that it is indisputable that TCM can treat virulent infectious diseases and SARS is not the most virulent one, why haven't we achieved a satisfactory result? It is people who glorify the theory, not the other way around. Even the best medical theories need to be practiced by doctors. It's known to all that now TCM is not well inherited with few brilliant newcomers who are not defined by number but by their inner quality. How many young and middle-aged TCM doctors are there who can follow the rules of TCM, study and research the medical theories and apply them in treating disease and saving life? There is a weird phenomenon showed in clinical practice: some TCM doctors prescribe Chinese herbs according to the theories of modern medicine. To combine TCM and modern medicine is a nice wish and it's still in trial. In present stage, TCM and modern medicine may either function independently or work cooperatively. However, we have to realize that modern medicine is the branch of modern science while TCM is an indispensable part of traditional Chinese culture. Both of them are scientific. To combine them organically is not an easy job at all due to the significant cultural difference and simply patching them up may lose the essence of both. For instance, SARS is caused by virus and may reduce immunity, so it seems reasonable to prescribe the Chinese medicine of heat-clearing and detoxifying in order to combat virus and apply the Chinese medicine of sweet in flavor and warm in nature to elevating immunity. In fact, the ingredients of Chinese medicine are very complicated, which cannot be fully elucidated by modern pharmacology and thus the previously stated prescription cannot be supported by modern medicine. From the perspective of TCM, the previously stated prescription violates the rules of treating pestilence due to dampness-heat and deviates from the principles of formula. The result of this prescription is not hard to predict.

It is consoling to see some insightful doctors who face up to SARS fearlessly, strictly comply with TCM theories and treat patients. They are the hope of TCM.

Confronting the crisis, we are obliged to appeal that TCM should be applied in treating infectious disease and its theories be observed. Let those doctors who excel in the TCM theory of pestilence to guide clinical treatment and the magic result is sure to be witnessed, benefiting the whole world.

The outbreak and resolving of SARS expose a series of long existed problems in medical field, which merit afterthoughts of the related people. In the long run, we should leave pure TCM more freedom to develop while promoting development of the combination of TCM and modern medicine. It relates to education, research and clinical practice and requires a long time to readjust. But it involves the well-being of billion people and it's not too late to correct the mistake.

Culture and Knowledge

Edited by Friedrich G. Wallner

www.peterlang.de

Peter Lang · Internationaler Verlag der Wissenschaften

Kambiz Badie / Maryam Tayefeh Mahmoudi

Strangification: A New Paradigm in Knowledge Processing and Creation

Frankfurt am Main, Berlin, Bern, Bruxelles, New York, Oxford, Wien, 2007.
148 pp., num. fig. and tab.
Culture and Knowledge. Edited by Friedrich G. Wallner. Vol. 7
ISBN 978-3-631-55989-5 · pb. € 41.90*

Strangification, as the core strategy of Constructive Realism, seems to be a potential source for feeding the methodological aspects which are essential to the creation of novel artificial systems. Due to this, it is significant to see how far Strangification can contribute to issues such as knowledge processing and knowledge creation as central issues in many cognitive, systemics, and inter-disciplinary studies. Within this context, strangification is worth being considered as a new paradigm for knowledge processing & creation. This volume tries to show such a characteristic of strangification. Design, planning, assessment, fitting and concept creation have been selected as the major issues to support this demonstration.

Contents: Capabilities of strangification in knowledge processing and creation issues · Knowledge processing and creation in design, planning and assessment issues · Strangification and knowledge creation through fitting · Creating new scientific concepts · Prospects of using strangification as a key strategy for creating knowledge creation in organizations

Frankfurt am Main · Berlin · Bern · Bruxelles · New York · Oxford · Wien
Distribution: Verlag Peter Lang AG
Moosstr. 1, CH-2542 Pieterlen
Telefax 00 41 (0) 32 / 376 17 27

*The €-price includes German tax rate
Prices are subject to change without notice
Homepage http://www.peterlang.de